YOGA CURES

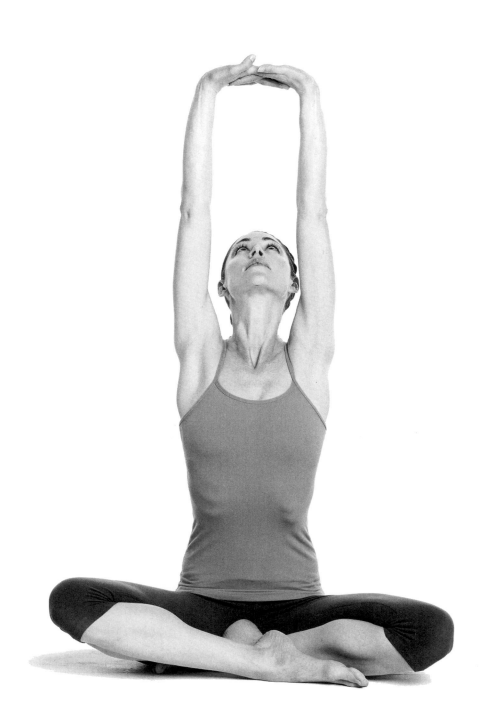

YOGA CURES

Simple Routines to Conquer
More Than 50 Common Ailments
and Live Pain-Free

TARA STILES

Author of *Slim Calm Sexy Yoga*

THREE RIVERS PRESS • NEW YORK

Library of Congress Cataloging-in-Publication Data
Stiles, Tara.
    Yoga cures : simple routines to conquer more than 50 common ailments and
live pain-free / by Tara Stiles; foreword by Deepak Chopra.
        p. cm.
1. Yoga. I. Title.
RA781.7.S754 2011
613.7'046—dc23
                                        2011034283

ISBN 978-0-307-95485-5
eISBN 978-0-307-95486-2

Printed in the United States of America

Book design by Lauren Dong
Interior and jacket photographs by Justin Borucki
Jacket design by Jessie Sayward Bright

10 9 8 7 6

First Edition

Contents

Bonus Material: Designing Your Own AT-HOME YOGA
RETREATS   174

Foreword by Deepak Chopra

Between work, raising a family, and coping with an uncertain economy, stress has become a "normal" part of daily life for most people. That could explain why so many Americans—about 16 million at latest count—have started taking yoga classes or doing yoga at home. For those seeking a lasting cure for anxiety or health issues and a greater sense of connectedness, yoga provides real and lasting benefits if they practice regularly. This ancient system connects mind and body through a series of postures, breathing exercises, and meditation. By stretching and toning the muscles, flexing the spine, and focusing the mind inward, yoga helps reduce stress. That can impact your overall health since stress plays at least some role in many illnesses. Studies show that chronic stress doubles the risk of heart attack, for instance.

Research into the health benefits of yoga is still in its infancy. But recent pilot studies point in promising directions. Yoga has been shown to lower blood pressure and heart rate, which can help reduce a person's risk of heart disease. There may be other heart benefits, too: a 2006 study found that yoga helped lower cholesterol levels and improve circulation in people who have cardiovascular disease. Some hospitals have incorporated yoga into their postcardiac rehabilitation programs.

While the evidence of yoga's success in reducing a person's body mass is mixed, one study did find that yoga can help people lose weight by leading them to a healthier lifestyle. The study reported that people who regularly practiced yoga started eating less, eating more slowly, and choosing healthier foods. They also showed fewer symptoms of eating disorders.

Many people report that yoga gives them an overall feeling of well-being. Research shows that it may also help alleviate specific kinds of pain, including migraine headaches, lower back problems, arthritis, and pain during childbirth. Researchers are not sure what mechanism is at work, but one theory is that the yoga postures work the way massage works. A yoga posture quickly sends the signal for "pressure" to the brain via myelinated (insulated) nerve fibers, while the signal for "pain" reaches the brain more slowly via less myelinated nerve fibers. The signal for "pressure" closes the receptor gate and shuts out the "pain" stimulus. Another theory is that yoga causes an increase in serotonin, the body's natural anti-pain chemical.

While more research is needed into these areas, people who practice yoga have also reported that they experience less insomnia and better digestive health. Pregnant women in particular seem to have an easier time sleeping when they do yoga. They are also less likely to develop high blood pressure or deliver prematurely.

Since yoga involves the mind as well as the body, it's not surprising that it may help reduce anxiety and depression, especially in people whose anxiety is related to an illness like cancer. A pilot study suggests that yoga may influence depression by increasing the alpha waves in the brain, which are associated with relaxation. Another possibility is that yoga reduces the amount of cortisol, a hormone that the body releases in response to stress. Some scientists think chronic high levels of cortisol may be tied to depression, as well as impaired immune function.

If the potential health benefits of yoga aren't enough to make you want to try it, consider this: Yoga can also make you look more toned and fit and help you move with greater ease, especially as you grow older. A 2007 study of the Hatha yoga style showed that it increased muscular strength, flexibility, and endurance. It's no wonder that many athletes use yoga to cross-train.

While yoga might not cure everything that ails you—or make your boss nicer—it will help you deal with stress better, and find your way more easily to feeling good in your life. And that can make a big difference in your overall health. So let's all take a big, deep breath and get started on your best path to overall health and happiness.

Introduction

Yoga brings you back to you . . . where all the good stuff is.

Anyone can do yoga and reap all its rewards. You don't need to be able to tie yourself into a pretzel or spend a year in silent devotion to gain all the amazing benefits of the practice. If you can breathe, you can do yoga. It's that simple. If you think you know yoga, or have never tried it because it seemed too woo-woo, chant-filled, mystical, and Om-centered (translate: OMG, I'm so bored!), then you should check out this book. Yoga is something both cooler and simpler, and it's fierce in what it can do for your life and health.

What do you really have to know to get started?

Inhale. Exhale. Repeat.

Don't let anyone fool you. It's not much harder than that. Once you rest your attention on your breath, everything else begins to open up with ease. There is no need to put a great, elevated authority between you and what you need. You can be your own great authority! I'm sure you've heard the old expression "Wherever you go, there you are." Well, it's true. So we might as well start to make where we are a great place to be!

Yoga can cure your body, settle your mind, and skyrocket your energy back to kindergarten levels! And if you're lifting an eyebrow and asking "Really?" just keep reading. How about being a ridiculously happy person with a super-healthy body and calm, focused mind? Yoga can cure everything from depression to anxiety; from old sports injuries and back pain to allergies, PMS, and even hangovers. I can't think of any reason why someone shouldn't at least try it, considering all of the incredible and practical benefits that come along with its regular practice. And that's what this book means to encompass: easy, fun cures using yoga in a fresh way to help alleviate or cure common complaints.

ZENSPIRATION

Imagine having your own personal room to breathe in that keeps expanding every time you practice. That's yoga.

Exhaustion cure? I've got it.

Suffering from "couch-stination" (a lack of desire to get off the couch)? Yep, that's here.

Feeling like the hunchback from hell after a week at the office? Your back is cramped, neck hurts, shoulders ache, and eyes burn? Check.

Suffering from desk fog (an overstressed, frazzled, and fried brain)? A few simple poses and deep breathing can help.

If you are in need of a little panic attack intervention, help for a droopy booty, saggy shoulders, mom-jean body, or bulging belly, or if you're suffering from "I can't touch my toes syndrome," there's something in here for you. But *Yoga Cures* covers the usual suspects as well: high blood pressure, colds, flu, vertigo, depression, thyroid imbalance, PMS, arthritis, and much more.

If you're feeling stretched to the limit, let these fifty-plus cures and the correlated routines unbind and de-stress you.

A LITTLE ABOUT ME

I've always been a goofball, tomboy, hippie girl who is much more comfortable in sweatpants and a hoodie than in fancy yoga gear. I don't like to think of myself as a yoga teacher, because it sets up a student/teacher thing that makes me feel like I need a ruler and a notebook to strut around the room. I prefer "yoga guide." I can help you get plugged in, but you don't owe me anything. No pledge of allegiance or donating your firstborn children. Nope. Just do the work. Be healthy and happy. That's cool enough for me. At the end of the day, you are your best teacher. I am just simply here to ride shotgun on your journey back to yourself.

My aim is to connect you back to you, where you'll find all the intuition you'll need to help you achieve your potential and live a healthy, inspired, creative, and joyful life. A yoga teacher once told me that she thought it was useful and great that I connect with the "Average Joe." That statement illustrates one of the main problems with how yoga has evolved. The problem with that thinking is that we are not separate from the Average Joe. In fact, we all are the Average Joe.

I've never thought of myself in any other way than interconnected with everyone on this planet. I depend on you. You depend on me. We are all connected and that's just how it is. Nothing woo-woo or out there about it. That's just nature. When we ignore the laws of nature we get out of balance. When we operate in harmony with nature we feel connected and in a state of flow, where everything starts to click and make sense. When we give over our power to others, yoga teacher or whomever, we stop following our own intuition and we disconnect from ourselves. Not good.

My life has taken me from country hippie girl to ballet dancer to Ford model. Then from there to YouTuber, blogger, and yoga studio owner. And now I am fortunate to call Deepak Chopra a friend, a teacher, and a student, and I am surrounded by many amazing people who are living out their dreams. If I can live my dream life, so can you.

If you were fortunate enough as a child you had at least one person who told you, "You can do anything you want with your life!" And hopefully as a grown-up, you've surrounded yourself with many people who cheer you on and support you in all your endeavors. If not, let me be that person. Any others along the way that tell you you'll never make it, well, they are only right if you let them be. Ultimately you're the only one holding yourself back or propelling yourself into your goals, desires, and dreams.

What does this have to do with yoga and yoga cures? Well, it's actually where the yoga comes in. You do the work. You get the results. The more you dive toward your goals, the more you'll realize the process is the ultimate destination. The great news is you start from right where you are, so you're already right where you need to be.

Often we spend our lives striving to decorate and improve our surroundings—a bigger house, a better car. We can spend our lives acquiring stuff with which to surround ourselves. But when we do yoga, we turn our attention inward and remember that our first home—our bodies and minds—needs to be dusted, remodeled, refreshed, and cared for if it is to remain strong. When we care for our inner world, our outer world reflects that care, and it also has a solid foundation from which to grow. Again, everything you need to know to build the life, health, and body you want is right there inside of you.

GET HAPPY, RIDICULOUSLY SO

We've all had moments where we feel absolutely fantastic. Better than fantastic, invincible. Cheesily happy and full of life. Maybe that feeling is now a distant childhood memory, or maybe that type of feeling happens sometimes, but not frequently and not commonly. When you do yoga regularly those ridiculously happy moments begin to happen more often, until they link together and become your life. Do you think I'm promising you too much? I'm not. We're all "wired" to have great capabilities, and that wiring can be enhanced based on how we live.

Your vagus nerve stretches from deep within the brainstem all the way into the belly. *Vagus* means wanderer. The nerve wanders through the body carrying impulses, winding its way up through the abdomen, diaphragm, and chest, up the neck outside the spinal cord, and into the brain. It's the literal stuff that makes up the mind/body connection. Vagus nerve stimulation therapy has been provided to epilepsy patients since 1997, using a pacemaker-like device implanted in their chests. It is being considered as a treatment for clinical depression as well. Fortunately, there is a noninvasive way to stimulate the vagus nerve and get our mind-body connection working up to speed. Ujjayi breathing in yoga, referred to often as Darth Vader breath, stimulates your vagus nerve, which literally sets off signals that make you happy. When you breathe deeply in yoga the vagus nerve sends messages between the central nervous system and the major organs; the hormone oxytocin is released, which helps us relax and reduces blood pressure and cortisol (aka stress) levels. We have our own ready-to-go anti-stress system within us at all times. We simply need to breathe deeply to access it.

We arrive in the world full of raw potential. Our life's work is either to deny this potential and hide under tension and fears, or strive to cultivate our individuality and refine our talents and see what we can make of ourselves.

I firmly believe that when enough people understand and experience the transformative and healing power of a regular yoga practice, we will become not only radiantly healthy as a culture, but more compassionate toward ourselves and others—happier, joyful, and full of life.

Ready to give it a try?

Yoga's Seven Big Benefits

Physical: The movements of yoga will carve out a long, lean, strong, and confident body.

Mental: All those deep breaths reset your mind back to its natural state: calm, focused, and sharp.

Psychological: All the focusing inward illuminates our behaviors and tendencies. The same habits we have on our mat are the ones we have in our lives. We see this, and we gain the freedom of choice. Who do I want to be? We get to create or re-create ourselves each day. Regular practice gives you a clear mind and the inspiration and courage to be constantly expanding and improving your life.

Neurological: When your brain is "on yoga" your neurological system is brought back into balance and is conditioned to steer you naturally toward a healthy lifestyle. Our bodies are constantly rewired to make whatever we practice get easier. When we practice healthy, balanced living we get more healthy, balanced living.

Intuitive: When there is tension in the body and mind, your intuition gets buried and your body switches to survival mode. Your yoga practice makes space in your body physically, releases tension, and calms your mind, making room for your intuition to float to the surface and guide you.

Creative: Creative juices start to flow when your body and mind begin to release mental blocks. Creativity doesn't like to come out when there are stressors, whether from physical tension or mental cloudiness. When the stress melts away, creativity can come out to play.

Connected: Yoga is the practice of getting connected. However you choose to view your spirituality, when you practice yoga, you remember that we all are connected, here to help each other, and that we have so much potential when we are kind to others.

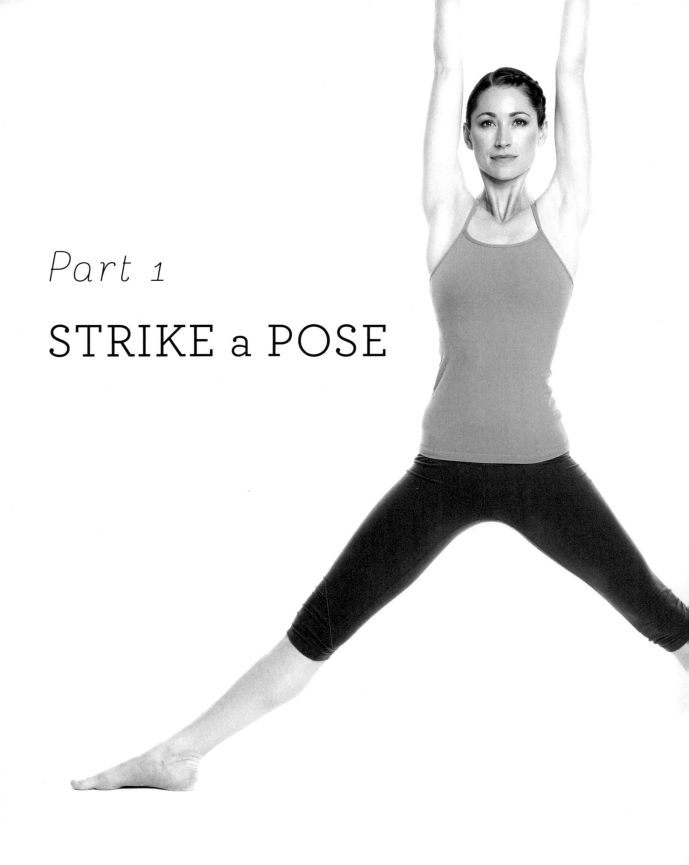

Part 1

STRIKE a POSE

ZENSPIRATION

There is no hurry. You have your whole life to practice, so enjoy being where you are right now. You're somewhere completely different each time you practice.

Yoga is made up of a series of fluid poses that are designed to heal your body and mind, with the breath guiding the way. Poses are rich with movement, whether the action is you flowing into the next pose, or breathing while remaining in one position. Your full, deep inhales and exhales bring the poses to life and connect you with your entire self.

When you breathe through the movement, things can flow with ease. The body can open and strengthen without resistance, and the mind will focus and settle. This quality of attention to the breath and calm awareness of movement separates the therapeutic power of yoga from other physical forms of movement, like sports, gymnastics, and dance.

Yoga is a moving meditation that unites the inner and outer you. Focusing on your breath is the core of any state of meditation. And it's true of yoga as well. Nothing is static or stuck in yoga.

A proper approach to physical alignment of the body is important for safety and therapeutic purposes, but making an extreme shape is not the goal. When you move with your breath, your body will tell you where it is ready to go, and you'll be at ease enough not to push or force it to move beyond that point. With yoga you start where you are, and you're somewhere different every day.

Chapter 1

What Is Yoga?

*You are not
just a drop
in the ocean,
you are the
mighty ocean
in the drop.
—Rumi*

Yoga means union. The Sanskrit word *yoga* has many meanings: to unite, to join, to contemplate, and to be absorbed. When we practice it regularly, we unite our mind, body, and spirit. We connect with ourselves, and we are able to connect more meaningfully with others and the world we are in. It's like calling a meeting with your whole self so that you can check in on you.

Yoga is the ultimate act of self-study. It is a daily dive deep into ourselves, where we come back refreshed and ready for all comers. Yoga goes much deeper than stretching. How you live in your body, how you experience it, is how you live in your mind, and the other way around, too. What do I mean by this? If your mind is tense your body is tense, and it dominos through the rest of your life. If your mind is out of balance, your body is out of balance, and your life can spiral out of control. If your mind is calm, open, and focused, your body and life also reflect and expand accordingly.

Yoga shows us how to wrangle the mind to serve us throughout our lives. Without such wrangling, the mind can spin off in many destructive directions. But get that monkey mind in hand, and your potential is limitless. Boundaries fade and life expands . . . the more you practice.

Why believe me? I'm not the only one to expound on the benefits of yoga. Many researchers throughout the world have studied yoga and meditation. They've just firmed up what we who do it already know: a regular yoga practice reduces stress, calms the mind, makes you happier, eases pain, increases mental sharpness, and prevents and heals all kinds of ailments and diseases. Yoga is a practice for living a better life, one deep breath at a time.

A BRIEF HISTORY OF YOGA—VERY BRIEF

No one knows exactly when the practice of yoga began, which makes sense since it is something that exists always and is inside of all of us. Traditionally, yoga is a practice to unite with the Absolute, recognizing that the Absolute is within all of us. Yoga joins together the body, mind, and spirit as one. Like air, water, and earth, yoga is an element that is contained in all of us. In the Indus Valley of northwestern India, stone carvings depicting figures in yoga poses have been found dating back five thousand years or more. There is a common misconception that yoga developed out of Hinduism. However, Hinduism's religious structures evolved much later and incorporated practices and ideas that are yoga traditions. Yoga probably arrived in the United States in the late 1800s, but it did not become widely known until the 1960s, when it became popular in the entertainment, pop culture, hippie, and intellectual scenes. George Harrison's interest in Eastern mysticism was sparked upon meeting with Swami Vishnu-devananda, the founder of Sivananda Yoga centers around the world, who handed Harrison a copy of his book *The Illustrated Book of Yoga* while the Beatles were on location in the Bahamas filming *Help!* The Beatles began to study Transcendental Meditation with Maharishi Mahesh Yogi in London and Wales, and eventually at his ashram in Rishikesh in the Himalayas. The Beatles were joined by Mia Farrow, Donovan, and Mike Love of the Beach Boys, who all jumped on the bandwagon.

Around the same time, Harvard professor Richard Alpert, now known as Ram Dass, conducted meditation and psychedelic experiments on prisoners. Upon being asked to leave Harvard for his unorthodox experiments, Alpert went to India to be with Neem Karoli Baba, who would become his guru and give him the name Ram Dass, meaning servant of Lord Rama. Yogis Sri Krishnamacharya, Swami Sivananda, Shri Yogendra, and Swami Kuvalayananda made efforts to include women and foreigners, who had been excluded from the practice. They also believed that Indian philosophy could coexist with Western science and medicine, an innovative idea that carries into the present. Swami Satchidananda, one of Sivananda's students, demonstrated yoga at Woodstock. The practice of yoga spread even deeper into the West when the influential B.K.S. Iyengar began his teacher/student relationship with the famous violinist

Yehudi Menuhin in 1954. Today, over $6 billion a year is spent on yoga, and approximately 15 million people in the United States are practicing. There are many styles, and hybrid styles, of yoga practice.

The poses are designed to heal you from the inside out. Each pose has specific purposes and benefits ranging from improving circulation, regulating digestion, enhancing metabolism, and improving range of motion to control, balance, and more. The yoga poses will carve out an optimal functioning body and mind. They will strengthen, lengthen, and shape your muscles in the best way to operate your entire system. An added bonus is that your body will be energized, strong, lean, and toned. Your skin will be glowing and fresh with life. The poses, in short, are designed to build your body's energy stores from the inside out. Unfortunately the history of yoga hasn't been immune to setbacks, misunderstandings, and corruption. Turned off by false gurus, religious overtones, attempted ownership, aggressive styles, and rigid prerequisites, many people have been excluded from the massive benefits of a practice that is a gift to everyone.

Patanjali was a sage and a scholar who compiled one of the earliest texts on yoga, called the Yoga Sutras. The Sutras could have been written as early as the first or second century BC or as late as the fifth century AD, exact dates are unknown. In the text, he outlined the Yamas and Niyamas, which together made up an ethical code of conduct for yogis to observe. Before we look at his code, I want to pause for a moment to focus on one aspect of it: ahimsa. It is an observance in the Yamas that calls for one to practice nonviolence. It's a practice in kindness to all living things, including ourselves.

Yoga is about recognizing and being good to ourselves from the inside out. Don't confuse being good to yourself with being selfish. We cannot extend love to others unless we truly love ourselves. If we are constantly hard on and judging ourselves, we do the same to others. We extend to others how we feel about ourselves. An easy way to see how we are treating ourselves is to look to those around us. They are a reflection of what's going on with us.

Hopefully, we have all treated ourselves well at times and have enjoyed how good that feels. The more we practice yoga, the better we feel, and the better we are able to cultivate a lasting attitude of kindness. This sets us up for a whole lot more ease in all areas of our lives.

THE EIGHT LIMBS OF YOGA

Patanjali wrote about the system known as Ashtanga Yoga, or the eight limbs of yoga. Here are the ethical guidelines he developed to be followed by any practitioner of yoga, including you, if you're so inclined:

1. Yama: Restraint, which lets us refrain from violence, lying, and stealing.

2. Niyama: Observances. Following a set of outlined rules that lead to contentment, purity, and tolerance.

3. Asana: The physical exercises (yoga poses).

4. Pranayama: The breathing techniques.

5. Pratyahara: The preparation for meditation, a withdrawal of the mind from the senses.

6. Dharana: A state of concentration and being able to hold the mind on one object for a specific time.

7. Dhyana: The act of meditation, the ability to focus on nothing, or no objects, indefinitely.

8. Samadhi: Absorption. Being present, and the realization of the essential nature of the self.

I believe that when the number of people practicing yoga reaches a critical mass, many of our collective mental and physical health problems will begin to fade away. But for yoga to really go mainstream people need to understand that its practice is something anyone can do.

You don't have to follow Patanjali's eight-limbed path, or move away to an ashram to have yoga benefit your life. You just have to begin to practice it. Simple. Easy. Powerful.

What do you do first? Breathe.

What next? Observe.

OBSERVE WITHOUT JUDGMENT

Observation without judgment is the basis for all meditation including yoga, which after all is simply a moving meditation. Yoga becomes truly useful when you can translate this attention and observation into all areas of your life. Otherwise, it would just be a lot of stretching and bending, which is fine and good, but not really the point.

You are the same person whether you're on the yoga mat or off of it. Practicing yoga is a great opportunity to observe your habits and tendencies. Do you give up too easily? Work too hard, but not effectively? Get down on yourself when things don't work out? Show off when things are going well? When we practice yoga we are giving ourselves the space to observe all this without judgment, to gain perspective, and cultivate positive, lasting change.

When we practice observing without judgment, we are giving ourselves the space and time to remove ourselves from the stresses of getting emotionally involved in the moment and simultaneously softening the desire to react solely on impulse. This will decrease stress and unwind tension at its source. Increased stress and anxiety can raise blood pressure, affect the immune system, and over time can promote sickness and disease. Good thing those long, deep breaths are available to rush in and save the day!

BALANCING ACT: BEING HERE, NOW

When you are balancing perfectly in a tree pose, everything is easy; your breath is deep and relaxed, and your muscles are working for you just as

In meditation we can watch the itch instead of scratching it.
—Ram Dass

you'd like. It's pure and simple. Efficient. When you are having a great day, the same things occur. Your breathing is relaxed, your body is working harmoniously with your mind; everything just feels easier because you are in a state of balance.

Why is balance important? From a life lesson standpoint, it's about learning to enjoy yourself without getting the ego involved. Say you're doing a headstand. The moment you think to yourself, "Wow, I'm doing this pose!" is usually the moment you'll topple out of it. You take yourself out of the moment and knock yourself off balance when you judge and think about what you are doing, rather than experiencing and enjoying what you are doing.

That's what yoga teaches. How to be fully present now, no matter the circumstance. We focus on breathing because each inhale creates more space in our bodies. We focus on movement, as each movement reminds us that every moment invites a new opportunity for change. Each exhale allows us to let go of the moment that has just passed. Our attention to each breath keeps us in the now.

Learning to savor the moment keeps us from living in constant worry and fear and tension over things that haven't happened yet and may never come to pass. Practicing yoga helps us to undo these bad mental habits and stress triggers that we often unknowingly pick up along the way.

But you might be asking, "What if the now is crappy? How can living in the moment help that?" When your life is not in balance and you're struggling to achieve stability, practicing observation without judgment gets really interesting . . . and very useful. How? Because you can learn to distance yourself from the roller-coaster ride of your emotions and circumstances but still enjoy the ride of life.

Outside means of escape like alcohol, drug use, and even overeating are a means of pushing uncertainty away and covering it up temporarily. And they may feel comforting for a moment, but I don't need to tell you that eventually they will cause more trouble than they ever solve. There is a big lesson in experiencing uncertainty and calamity with a sober focus. The most chaotic moments are the ones from which we can learn the most. Let's go back to tree pose. When your tree pose is going crazy and you're falling, and your leg is burning, and it feels impossible to maintain any sort of stability, practice observing what's happening instead of getting wrapped up in the circumstance. If you can learn to be easy with your breath in these moments, your body and mind will follow.

All the body's systems and processes—your nerves, your emotions—take instruction from what is going on with your breath. When your breathing is easy and deep, your body works efficiently and your mind settles. That doesn't mean that your balance (in tree pose or anywhere else) will be perfect and your life will be seamless, but you'll be better equipped to deal with the wobbles and earthquakes that get thrown into the mix.

You can fall out of a tree pose with ease, or with frustration and a sense of defeat. Just like you can take a spill in your life and decide to dust yourself off—with a chuckle or an annoyed grunt—and get back up, or you can stay down, lie there, and give up. It's entirely up to you. It's your life . . . and your practice. And as I said before, what you practice on the mat is what you end up doing in your life.

Any of the yoga poses could be substituted in this analogy. How you practice is much more meaningful than what yoga moves you can or cannot do. A successful tree pose probably won't change your life. Learning how to keep your breath easy, long, and deep no matter what the circumstance? It absolutely will.

FIND YOUR MEANING

I'm going to challenge you over and over to imagine yoga as moving beyond the poses and even the breath. I'd like to persuade you to expand your idea of what yoga can do for you beyond deep breaths, down dogs, and feeling great, although yoga is also about all of the above. What if you could be practicing and enjoying all the benefits of yoga and meditation at every moment during your entire life? Imagine having an extra split second to make decisions, more space inside your body and mind, and the ability to feel energized, creative, strong, open, and inspired all day long.

The more often we check in, or tune in, the more we feel connected, the healthier our bodies and minds get, and the more inspired and aware we become. It's like juicing up a rechargeable lightbulb with no limit to the brightness and quality of the bulb. You are the bulb. Your yoga is the current. Your possibilities are endless.

Try it now. Stop whatever you are doing just for a moment. Close your eyes and draw your attention inward. Begin to observe without getting involved. Watch sensations as they come and go. Do this for one minute, three times a day. You'll enjoy a calm sense of ease.

When you are in the state of flow, you come into balance and experience happiness, health, and joy. The practice of yoga is designed to keep you in the state of flow so you can experience health, happiness, and joy during your entire life. The practice of yoga clears the clutter that collects on you like dust during each day. The practice of yoga brings you back to remembering your true nature, back to happiness, health, and joy. You didn't arrive in this world full of worries. Yoga shows you how to dissolve anything that is blocking you from living out your full potential.

Yoga is on your side big-time!

DISCOVERING YOUR YOGA

Yoga was discovered, not invented, the same as water and fire. You can't experience water until you drink a glass. Same with yoga. When you practice it, you get it. When you do yoga you feel incredibly fantastic. When you do it consistently for a long time you feel invincible, like a superhero. Over the years, as with many traditions and systems that make people feel good (often religions), people have built complicated layers on top of yoga, putting themselves in positions of power as gatekeepers to secrets. This tends to corrupt people, as well as muddle the traditions themselves.

In many ancient traditions, yoga has been passed down from guru to disciple. The guru is someone who has gained understanding and is living the experience of yoga. The student comes to the guru for guidance. Any good guru will always point you back to yourself, point you inward.

Yoga is available to everyone. We all are our own masters. And we all have what we need to be healthy and happy inside of us. We have to get plugged into that today—not by copying what an old guru said we should do, but by doing yoga. Period. Proper guidance and teachers are helpful, but your best teacher is yourself. All the answers are right there inside.

Your yoga practice should ground you and bring out the best in you. The practice of yoga isn't meant to take you out of or away from your life. You don't have to live out some idea of yoga that might be floating around from the past; you don't have to live someone else's yoga. You don't have to change your name to something Sanskrit, adopt a new identity, and isolate yourself in an ashram to live your yoga. Your yoga practice is there to ground you and bring out the best in you for your entire life, beginning exactly where you are now.

TIME TO MAKE THE YOGA

All of the yoga poses have been designed and refined to serve the needs of the body and mind. Yoga is an ever-evolving practice that you can tailor to your own needs and requirements. We have different needs than yogis thousands of years ago did. Ancient yogis never had to deal with carpal tunnel syndrome, frazzled eyes from computer screens, and tight hips from sitting at desks all day. They seemed to be on to something by practicing regular meditation and feeling at peace in the world.

Yoga works. It can cure us when we stay at ease in our bodies, and follow our breath. It doesn't work by pushing or forcing poses to happen. There are so many variations and options within the poses that you can stay where you are and never worry about forcing your body to do something that doesn't feel right. When practicing yoga you will feel your muscles working and your mind focusing, but you should be able to stay relaxed and at ease during the entire practice.

Practicing being at ease is much more useful than practicing frustration. When something frustrates or presents itself as a major block, simply back off, wait for your breath to return to a long and deep rhythm, then come back to what you are doing.

If a door is open, walk through. If it is closed, knock and wait a few breaths. If it stays closed, you can return another day. When you practice with ease, eventually things aren't as challenging because you have changed your approach. If you muscle through a pose you might achieve the shape of the pose, but in terms of your energy you'll be a wound-up ball of stress with high blood pressure, a tense mind that can't focus, and a body so tight that it can't move. It's a mistake to believe that forcing is better than easing your way into a pose . . . or into life for that matter. When you move with ease, you'll be at ease. You'll get more done with less effort. You'll get further faster. It's a mirage to believe that tension and agitated striving is the way.

What else do you need to know before you begin? You know to breathe, observe, ease into it . . . but how? Where do you "put" your body during all this? That's up next.

THE LINE STARTS HERE: ESSENTIAL ALIGNMENT

There are a few simple alignment tips that can be useful in your practice. With them in mind, you can experience yoga fully and have a good time without injury.

Always Favor Backing Off Rather Than Pushing

Though I just said it, it bears repeating: take it easy. You should always be able to carry on a casual conversation during yoga. (Not that you should talk to your neighbors during yoga class, but the state of your breath should be easy and not strained.) When you feel your breath getting forced and shortened, back out of the pose, or rest until you can breathe deeply again. Child's pose is a great place to take a breather.

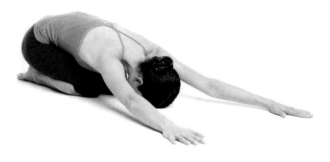

CHILD'S POSE

Gently come onto all fours. Relax your hips and sit back on your heels. Rest your forehead on the ground and breathe deeply into your back. Stay here for five long, deep breaths.

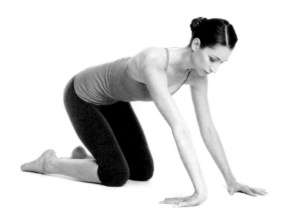

HEALTHY AND SUPPORTED WRISTS
Hands and Knees Wrist Release

A lot of yoga poses are spent bearing weight on your arms, get into the habit of warming up your wrists before you practice to avoid pain and injury. If you spend a lot of time working at a computer it's good to do this exercise daily to maintain healthy wrists. When you are practicing, spread the fingers wide like you are digging into wet sand. You want to give your hands a strong and steady foundation.

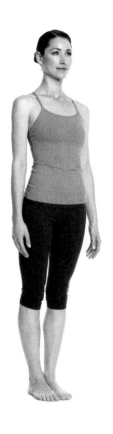

FIND YOUR FEET
Standing

Your feet are your foundation in a lot of the poses. Make sure you stand firm on them! Stand at the top of your yoga mat. Feet are parallel and slightly apart, under your hip bones. Your hip bones aren't at the outside of your hips so make sure your feet aren't too far apart. You can check by placing two fists between your feet. That's about the width of your hip bones. Close your eyes and bring your attention to your breath. Lengthen and deepen your inhales and exhales and continue breathing at this nice, slow pace for five full breaths. Gently open your eyes.

KNEES OVER TOES
Warrior 2

This alignment rule is good for the health of your knees and other joints. In warrior poses and most standing poses you want to make sure your knees are over your ankles, not rolling in or out, or moving past your toes. You may not feel strain in your knees right away if you compromise your alignment, but over time misalignment causes wear and tear. So make sure to always check the alignment of your knees over your ankles.

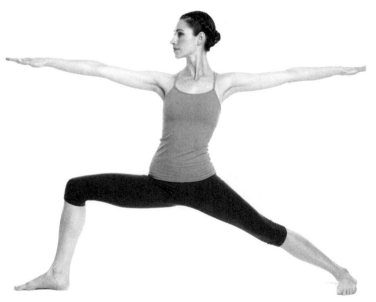

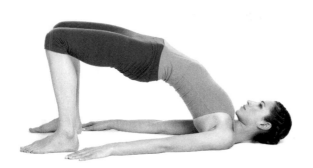

LENGTHEN THE SPINE
Bridge

Yoga is about creating space in the body. Most poses involve the spine whether they are forward bending, twisting, or back bending. Always consider creating more space between each vertebra and the next, rather than rounding and crunching the spine. When arching, the tailbone is rooted down and the chest lifted. Try to avoid crunching and sinking into the lower back. Make sure to extend evenly through your entire spine, from the back of your neck through your tailbone. Lengthening the spine will ward away a lot of back problems.

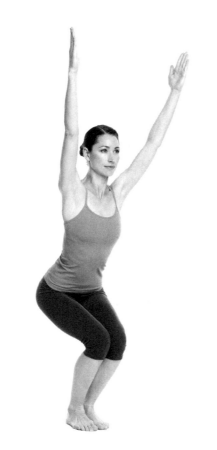

DON'T GRIP YOUR MUSCLES
Chair

Your muscles will do what they need to do to be in a pose. There is no need to grip your muscles to hold a position. Engage the muscles that you need for each pose and rest what you don't need. You'll find your body can work much more efficiently when you avoid gripping and flexing your muscles while moving. And don't worry, you are still getting all the workout you'll need. No flexing required.

Always Remember to Breathe

After you've gotten your alignment down, don't forget to come back to the breath and feel each pose and movement. When you are this focused on the breath, it becomes the guiding yoga pose. All the movements come out of the breath like a wave. Your body takes on a lightness and a sense of efficiency and ease and your mind calms. Whenever you lose track of the breath, simply guide your attention back. The breath will always be there waiting for you to follow it.

A good guideline for breathing is to expand, lengthen, and strengthen your body with each breath in, and release, ease, and relax your body with every breath out. Moving through challenges becomes far easier when you can get your breath working for you this way. To have lasting strength, we need to begin by embodying flexibility. When we hold our breath we tense. The body becomes stiff, the mind goes into frazzled mode, and things can spiral out of control. Deep breaths allow the body to work efficiently, the mind to focus in a calm way. When you hold your breath and attempt to push through the movements, not much happens except a lot of forcing, building up tension and stress that can lead to a habit of forcing and injury. When you breathe with ease the poses happen smoothly, and when they don't you learn the needed patience that allows you to breathe through the tension.

What else do you need to remember before you get started? It's all about taking CARE . . .

TAKE "CARE" OF YOURSELF; THE YOGA WILL FOLLOW

If you have clarity, attention, relaxation, and ease, you'll be on your way to feeling great with yoga. Remembering these four qualities, remembering to CARE, can help you through your practice every step of the way.

Clarity. Know what you are doing and why. Are you practicing to heal from a specific ailment, to de-stress, or something else? Your reasons might change daily, but considering what they are is useful. Forming an intention and approaching your practice with clarity will get you started—and keep you pointed—in the right direction.

Attention. By now you know, attention is the foundation of yoga. Keeping your attention on your breath during meditation and yoga (moving meditation) takes practice. Whenever your attention wanders, just simply guide it back.

Relaxation. It's interesting that we have to learn how to relax. We spend a lot of our lives tensing up in preparation to "do battle" each day, with our families, bosses, or our to-do list. When we release the tension, step away from the fray, we have more room in our bodies and minds. And yes, again, it's all in your breathing. Deep, attended breaths lead directly to relaxation.

Ease. Finding an ease in your body and mind is essential in yoga. When your breathing gets shorter and faster, know that you can always bring it back to full and deep. Again, your body and mind will follow your breath. So control it, rather than the other way around. And again, you don't "grip" it, you just attend to it . . . the lungs will open up all on their own.

Want to find out what else yoga can help with when practiced regularly? Check out the next chapter: it's a look at the science and at some real people who've been helped by doing yoga. Do you need to read it before doing the cures? No . . . and yes. No, because the poses work when you do them. Period. Yes, because with a clear understanding of why you are doing anything, you get more, you get further, and you get there faster.

THE POCKET YOGA GUIDE: Five Steps to Always Remember

Step 1. Become an observer
It's quite interesting to step outside and watch yourself. You will learn something new every time. Observing your actions takes you out of reacting mode. You gain more time to see what's going on and adjust accordingly.

Step 2. Watch, don't judge
While doing this, remember not to judge. You can learn a lot more about your habits and behaviors if you can simply observe without judgment. This doesn't mean you abandon all ability to discern good from not good! It just means you get to take a break from instant reactivity, just to watch.

Step 3. Wait
The reason it's called practice is because it requires practice. Every day you keep at it. At first, it may not seem like much of anything is happening. But if you keep at it your body will open and strengthen and your mind will calm and settle. Have patience with yourself. Yoga doesn't always work on the schedule you may want it to. Allow time for its lessons to simmer. Enjoy the process. Remember life is a work in progress and you're always right in the middle of it . . . so that progress is sometimes hard to see.

Step 4. Keep it up
If you feel like giving up, because nothing good seems to be happening, keep practicing. Things are changing in your body and mind. Trust the process. Trust yourself. Neither will let you down.

Step 5. Don't worry
There is nothing to worry about. You are right where you need to be and you have all the tools you need.

When you calm your mind, everything opens up. Stress melts away, worries dissolve, the body gets crazy healthy, and your energy levels skyrocket. The only thing standing in your way is your own limited thinking about yourself. Remember what I said earlier? That you have it all within you? You do. Always. You just need to quiet down and really listen.

Chapter 2

The Mind/Body Connection and the Science Behind How Yoga Cures

You might have had the experience of being in a grumpy mood before a yoga class, then you walk out feeling like a completely different person, happy as can be. What's happening? Meditation and yoga can actually change your brain on a cellular level. Today we have some interesting science that is explaining how yoga does this and how yoga cures. In this chapter, I'll share just a little of the coolest research I found about the "why." A lot of it has to do with the control we have over our bodies, minds, and even our genes when practicing yoga.

MAKE LIKE A MONK

Scientists studied eight Tibetan Buddhist monks who had put in at least ten thousand hours of practice in compassion meditation. Using a brain scan called functional magnetic resonance imaging, the researchers pinpointed regions that were active during compassion meditation. In almost every case, the monks had more enhanced activity in these regions of the brain than novices used as controls. Activity in the left prefrontal cortex (believed to be the seat of positive emotions such as happiness) swamped activity in the right (site of negative emotions and anxiety). If you're scratching your head a bit over this, it means, in short: the monks were happier, their brains were happier. And a happier brain means a healthier one. It means a healthier body, too.

This study got a lot of scientists excited about the capabilities of our brains because it showed that the brain has neuroplasticity (or in other words is pliable, and shapable). The brain is able to change its structure and function by expanding or strengthening the circuits that are used, and shrinking or weakening those that are rarely engaged. We can actually change and improve our state of mind and our brains through yoga; the more we practice the better we feel.

STUCK WITH YOUR GENES?

Many scientists are also focusing lately on epigenetics, the study of the molecular mechanisms by which the environment controls gene activity. What does this mean to us? They are discovering the power of the mind/body connection, or what yogis have been up to throughout the ages. For generations, we grew up being told that we're stuck with what we're born with. That we're a product of our genes. Whether it be the skinny gene, the fat gene, the cancer gene, or the diabetes gene, we were told that whatever health issues our parents or grandparents or other generations had, we too would share them. Now, through the science of epigenetics, we are learning that it is much more complicated than that. To say we are solely a product of our genes is just not true at all.

The good news: it's not so much about the genes you're born with, but about how you communicate with your genes through your lifestyle, diet, and environment. It makes a lot of sense, actually, that we are able to change at a genetic level, seeing that we are living, breathing, changing beings, not statues made of stone. Several studies have now shown that changing lifestyle factors cause changes in gene expression. Stress, toxins, and negative behaviors activate chemical switches that turn genes on and off; the reverse is true, too. And guess what practice reduces stress and toxins and negative health behaviors? Yep, you guessed it: yoga. But that's not all. According to Dr. Frank Lipman, founder and director of the Eleven Wellness Center in New York City and a pioneer in the fields of inte-

Go GABA!

Researchers at Boston University School of Medicine found that for experienced yoga practitioners, brain levels of GABA increased by 27 percent after a session of yoga. GABA is one of our brain's four primary neurotransmitters. It works to reduce stress and anxiety, as well as regulate the other neurotransmitters. This suggests that the practice of yoga should be explored as a treatment for disorders associated with low GABA levels, such as depression and anxiety. These results also explain that post-yoga happy feeling that comes after an hour or so of doing it.

grative and functional medicine, "Bathing your genes in the right environment [in terms of your nutrition, emotions, and thoughts] will turn the genes for health on and the 'disease' genes off." Your genes are controlled by "coding" that tells them to be expressed or not expressed—and researchers believe that this expression can be almost completely controlled by your environment and lifestyle. Also, the way you practice expressing your genes during your life will be passed down to your children. It's called epigenetic inheritance.

In short, we are much more responsible for our actions and behaviors, and their outcomes, than we might have thought previously! This is both heartening and perhaps a little frightening because we can't push the blame onto somebody else. But isn't it better to be in control than to feel like a puppet controlled by your family genes?

Now that we know we have the ability to change our genes, our brains, and our entire lives, how do we go about it? I know you already know my answer, and you've seen just a glimpse of the science that supports it: yoga. Committing yourself to a regular yoga practice is one of the best things you can do for yourself—and your children and grandchildren—during your lifetime!

Yoga teaches us how to be easy in our own skin. We learn how to use our bodies effectively, while we wash off the daily stresses of life before they collect within us to do their damage. We learn to relax and focus our minds so we can concentrate on our tasks fully when necessary and relax fully when we'd like. Less stress means better choices in general, as the happier you are the less you "need" to reach for comfort from the wrong places. But more on that later.

SIMPLE CURE, POWERFUL POSSIBILITIES

It's quite simple. Yoga cures. But you have to practice it regularly, at least three to four times a week, for it to work for you. Once you make it a habit, you'll notice a desire to practice every day, even if that means ten minutes of meditation one day, an hour of physical yoga the next. What and how long you practice will vary, but consistency is essential.

Mind/body medicine has shifted from an underutilized fringe movement to a regular supplement to traditional Western medical care. It is now more commonly referred to as integrative medicine, and is an approach aimed at treating the whole person. Integrative medicine, a marriage of alternative and conventional medicine, is key to remedying our collectively poor state of health. Interestingly, approaches that had been categorized as alternative, such as Chinese, Tibetan, and ayurvedic medicines, massage therapy, homeopathy, meditation, and yoga, all predated conventional Western medicine by thousands of years. There is something to be said for older and wiser when developing and advancing health practices. The integrative approach builds a bridge between the conventional and alternative to find a workable solution, while still maintaining the integrity of each method.

Observation without judgment, the founding element of both yoga and science, marries the two disciplines into a sustainable, healing approach. Often the correct answer is the most obvious one. Dueling banjos can conflict and compete to invalidate each other's importance, or collaborate to make lovely music. Often a battle can be won by joining forces. The battle of getting our health out of the gutter is one worth fighting. Even better, using an approach of ease and relaxation, you can dissolve disease and change your genes and your fate, replacing chronic ailments with a long life, one filled with health, happiness, and vitality.

MIND ~~OVER~~ IS MATTER

We all have heard or used the phrase "mind over matter." It's often used when we are trying to get through a challenging circumstance. The practice of yoga shows us that our minds and our bodies are not only connected, they are interconnected and affect each other in very intricate ways that science has only begun to explore, let alone explain. But you can experience the mind/body interconnection through yoga.

You can shift your state of body and mind through yoga. You can even get very specific and tailor your practice to meet the needs of your life, even the needs of each day and moment. For example, if you feel anxious or nervous about an upcoming event, calming techniques like alternate nostril breathing and some simple seated side and forward bends will help balance your nervous system, calm your mind, and dissolve anxiety with each inhale and exhale.

Even a simple variation in hand position during meditation can help. Want an extra boost of energy? Try meditating with your palms facing up on your thighs. Need some grounding? Place your palms down.

If you feel groggy or a little fuzzy and unfocused, some yoga poses targeted at increasing blood flow, like headstands and twists, followed by meditation, can sharpen your focus and give you a nice side-effect-free boost of energy. If you need to lose weight, a regular yoga practice will reprogram your mind to actually crave foods that are healthy for you. Practicing shoulder stands at least once a day will regulate the thyroid gland, which controls your metabolism. The pose also calms the mind, which helps reduce anxious and compulsive behaviors, including overeating. A regular yoga practice is the real deal for radiant health. Its cures are endless.

Each person has a unique and individual experience with every practice. That's why I feel that telling someone what they should be feeling isn't one of the best ways to teach and share yoga. It is our own feelings—our intuition, awareness, and personal power—that lead the way to healing. I won't instruct you how to feel, but I will lead you to specific techniques that connect you back to yourself. The answers will come to you when you are on the right path.

What else can yoga cure . . . well, most everything!

YOGA CURES: CHRONIC DISEASE

In 2007 Kyeongra Yang of the University of Pittsburgh School of Nursing published an article in the journal *Evidence-Based Complementary and Alternative Medicine* reviewing published studies on the use of yoga to reduce obesity, high blood pressure, high glucose levels, and high cholesterol—major risk factors for illnesses including heart disease, stroke, and diabetes. The studies Kang reviewed found that a regular yoga practice lowers body weight, blood pressure, cholesterol, glucose levels, and stress levels. Yoga promotes physical activity, a healthy diet, better mood, a feeling of self-efficacy, and an overall strong quality of life. The studies took a variety of yoga practices into consideration, including physical postures and meditation techniques.

It's no secret that a lot of research is funded by pharmaceutical companies. The quest: finding a very profitable golden-ticket drug that suppresses symptoms or cures diseases caused by unhealthy living. Often these drugs work and can be very useful in helping prolong life or suppress symptoms, but drugs also often have unpleasant and harmful side effects, and in themselves are rarely a complete cure.

Unlike drugs, yoga has no harmful side effects when practiced with attention and care. People may get injured from time to time in a yoga class, but this is most often because they aren't paying attention and are trying to force themselves in positions for which they aren't ready. The real heart of yoga is paying attention to exactly what is going on with you, and then acting accordingly.

We have a choice when it comes to how we live, and how we think about and promote our health and the health of the world. We can point fingers and blame the system for its unfair and corrupt practices. Or we can take charge of our own health and the health of those we care about by living a healthy life instead of relying on pills to fix things we may have been able to prevent in the first place. So instead of getting down on the system that we live in, where pharmaceutical companies sweep in with a magic pill to fix every problem, we can begin to change ourselves and our world . . . one breath at a time. The useful work is always within. Remember, it all happens by taking it one breath at a time.

YOGA CURES: BOOST YOUR MOOD

Yoga practice has profound effects on mood. I speak from experience when I tell you that you can be having a pretty bad day, or be in a bummer of a mood, head into a yoga class, and after an hour or so you'll be in a completely different and better state of mind. Regular practice has stabilized my mood, and moved everything in a positive direction.

It's not that yoga practice puts you into an emotional coma where you don't feel anything. It's quite the contrary. Yoga allows us to see things more clearly and gain room to move within our emotional lives. Yoga gives us the space to observe what we would like to do without getting wrapped up and consumed with the moment. The results of this balanced perspective can be tremendous in nearly every aspect of our lives. We are more productive about work when we are less emotionally involved, tense, and worried. We can cultivate lasting and meaningful relationships when we have a little space from our emotions and so are able to communicate with compassion, focus, and ease.

Australian researchers at Deakin University in Melbourne conducted a study using yoga as both a preventive therapy and a treatment for symptoms of mental illness. Participants went through a six-week yoga program that included breathing techniques, yoga poses designed to enhance strength, vitality, and flexibility, and guided relaxation and meditation. The aim was to see if participants would increase their resistance to emotional distress by developing greater calmness, self-acceptance, a more balanced perspective on life, and enhanced concentration—all things the researchers believed could potentially be gained from yoga. They compared symptoms of stress, anxiety, and depression across three groups: regular yoga practitioners, beginners practicing yoga as therapy for depression and stress for the first time, and a control group that did not practice yoga. The study also looked at the participants' sense of intrinsic spirituality (an inherent sense of spiritual connection or fullness) before and after the six-week yoga practice.

REAL-LIFE CURES: Dave's Obsessive-Compulsive Disorder (OCD)

Meet Dave, a Strala regular (one of the early adopters, from the time I led yoga classes out of my apartment). For quite some time, he suffered from OCD, an anxiety disorder in which a hyperactive mind finds often arbitrary obsessions and rituals to keep itself occupied. Those who have OCD relate that at times the brain feels a bit like a pinball machine: pinging from one subject to the next, out of control.

Dave says he has experienced a 60 to 70 percent improvement in his OCD symptoms over the last two years of sporadic yoga practice. Dave says he feels breathing and meditation are the activities that are most directly useful in slowing down his brain.

If you search online, like Dave did, for connections between OCD and yoga, you may find information on the benefits of meditation and alternate nostril breathing (a technique that is a huge cure for anxiety among other things), but likely not all that much on yoga's usefulness with this disorder. You will find a slew of medical sites, and a slew of medications available as the first suggested treatment for the disorder. What's the harm in giving yoga a try, like Dave did, and seeing if this "old school" treatment can't help?

When the three study groups were compared at the end of six weeks, the people in the beginners' yoga group on average had lower levels for symptoms of depression, anxiety, and stress than before the beginning of the study. The people who already practiced yoga and the people in the control group, not surprisingly, showed no change. In addition, the participants in the beginning yoga group showed growth in their self-reported level of spiritual connection.

YOGA CURES: ACHES AND PAINS

From day-to-day body aches that result from too much office or desk time—and neck, shoulder, hip, and wrist tension—to more chronic issues like back pain, sciatica, and sports injuries, or even problems caused by improperly practiced yoga, a regular yoga practice has improved symptoms and often reversed these conditions. Even arthritis and fibromyalgia and their resulting pain, discomfort, and decreased range of motion have been helped by yoga.

Scientists from Johns Hopkins University in Baltimore divided a group of thirty sedentary adults with rheumatoid arthritis (RA) into two groups: one participated in an eight-week program of yoga and the other was put on a wait list and served as the control. The people in the yoga group participated in two one-hour classes per week and were instructed to practice at home as well. Traditional yoga poses were modified as needed to accommodate any physical limitations from the disease. Also included in the sessions were deep breathing, relaxation, and meditation techniques. The research team found that those who participated in eight weeks of yoga had significantly fewer tender and swollen joints than they did before starting class. The wait-list group saw no significant changes.

James Carson, PhD, a researcher and psychologist at the Oregon Health and Science University in Portland, enlisted people suffering from fibromyalgia in a weekly two-hour yoga class and found that symptoms such as pain, fatigue, and stiffness were reduced by 30 percent in more than half of the participants. A control group continued their regular treatment regimen and reported no change in symptoms. Carson believes that the yoga program used in the study is a low-impact way for fibromyalgia patients to get moving, and performing yoga may even change the way the central nervous system responds to pain.

REAL-LIFE CURES: Heidi's Car Accident

Heidi Kristoffer, a yoga teacher, has healed her body's pretty dramatic trauma and limitations through yoga. She had suffered a herniated disc in her neck from a car accident, and for as long as she could remember, she thought she just had a bad back and that her back pain was normal. After a while Heidi started getting sciatica down her left side. This is when doctors discovered that she'd actually broken the L2 and L3 vertebrae in her spine. Because the fractures were not diagnosed, they didn't heal properly, and her doctors didn't think they ever would. One doctor told Heidi that he had never seen anyone with her injuries standing, much less moving around. One thing her doctors did agree on was that yoga was good for her back and had probably saved her from further injury.

Heidi has avoided surgery by building up the core muscles surrounding the spine that keep everything in place. The more she worked on strengthening and focused on alignment and on listening to her body, the stronger and healthier her back became. Now Heidi wakes up every day pain free, happy, and excited about life.

WHAT'S YOUR "FIX" GOING TO BE: YOU OR A PILL?

The stories I've included in this chapter are but a small handful of anecdotes from my studio; there are so many more. From a friend with MS who found help with the spasticity of her muscles to someone who claims that yoga even cured her psoriasis.

There is a pill to fix pretty much everything that goes wrong with your body or your mind. There is fast, cheap, addictive food available everywhere we look. There are diets that promise to shed excess pounds in days. There is workout equipment that promises to minimize physical effort while getting your body strong, lean, and toned. But none of these solutions are sustainable. In fact they lead you to ill health, not strength and wisdom. But yoga done properly is different.

When we do yoga we realize that we are one expansive, malleable unit: body, mind, and spirit are entirely ours to shape. From this realization, we can begin to approach our lives in a grounded, informed way that is useful for living a happier, healthier, and joy-filled life.

Since we cannot separate ourselves into mind and body, it is very useful to treat the entire person rather than individual parts. The cures you'll find on the following pages address your whole self. Your body and mind are interconnected, so it's important to address your entire self, instead of isolating problems and ailments. Sure, healing individual parts is useful when it comes to dealing with a cut finger or a broken bone, but when we get into more complex ailments like stress, insomnia, and depression, it's essential to take all of you into account. More and more Western-trained medical doctors are recommending yoga, meditation, and relaxation techniques to promote health, and also prevent and heal ailments and disease. I've seen a big shift over the time I've been teaching. People's doctors have sent them to yoga classes for a wide range of problems—everything from backache to anxiety, high blood pressure to obesity, and even to aid in things as serious as cancer.

You know now from this chapter's brief walk through the research that meditation, yoga, and other relaxation and visual techniques can serve as a great benefit to anyone who practices.

As I said before, science is finally catching up to what yoga practitioners have known for years: yoga has always been able to cure the body and mind. Yoga is something that belongs to all of us, so we all have the power to cure ourselves. The more research illustrates the healing power of yoga, the more opportunities our generation and the generations to come will have to access their own inner healer and enjoy a transformation into radiant health. Okay, let me step down from the pulpit here. I know this has gotten a little heady and preachy. But as I've just shown you, you don't have to believe me, trust the science and trust yourself. Your health will thank you for it.

Now you know you want to give it a try. Where to get started? Just turn the page . . . and follow your nose.

Chapter 3

To Get Started, Just Follow Your Nose

Thinking is useful in our everyday lives when we have to solve problems, make decisions, and cross the street. But to build the tools we need to heal ourselves—intuition, feeling, and self-awareness—we need to quiet our minds. The answer to doing so? It's right at the tip of your nose.

Often, we walk around mindless, muscling and forcing our way into and through things. When we start with the breath, we begin with the air we take in. More air means everything becomes lighter, easier, and more efficient, like a nice warm breeze blowing through your body's house.

When we learn to pay attention to our breathing, we end up bringing in a breath of fresh air to the rest of our lives, too. Life changes, expands, becomes easier, lighter, and more fun the more we bring in breath, space, light . . . air. Good stuff.

Breathing is something everyone must do to stay alive. Meditation is something that anyone can do to thrive. You can meditate for five seconds, five minutes, or an hour. Take as much or as little time as you have. Make time if you can. The benefits of meditation are astounding and range from feeling a sense of ease, to reducing stress, to creating focus, experiencing heightened creativity, and dissolving negative urges, as well as creating a powerful feeling of connectivity and purpose. Once you dive in and experience the benefits, hopefully you will make time often to return to the breath.

What is meditation? Simply, it's calming the mind by watching the breath, instead of tuning into our rapid-fire, worry-filled thoughts. And it is a powerful practice. It connects us to our core. The more we do it, the more we realize that everything we need is right there inside.

Something interesting happens when we go from someone who is breathing to someone who is watching the breath come and go. We click into observer mode. In the moment of switching to being mindful of our breaths, space begins to open up for our minds to calm. Our heartbeats slow down and we have room to breathe. Observation becomes meditation.

TIME TO MAKE THE YOGA: CATCHING YOUR BREATH

Let's go over a few things that happen with the breath, both when it's in control, and out of our control. We'll cover some techniques that are useful, whether you are practicing yoga, relaxing at home, or commuting to work.

Short, Fast, Out-of-Control Breathing

We've all experienced this type of breathing, whether we're racing up a flight of stairs, engaged in a heated argument, or hearing some exciting news. When your breathing becomes short and fast in yoga, that's a sign to back off with the physical stuff until you can lengthen and deepen your breath. Short and fast breathing happens, but when it does, take the time to guide it back.

Next time you race up a flight of stairs or are rushing to get somewhere, notice your breath. If it's short and fast, take a moment to bring it back to easy breathing. If you can keep coming back to easy, full breathing even when doing difficult things, this translates into all kinds of great benefits in the rest of your life.

Easy Breathing

Hopefully this is the quality of breath we have for most of the day when we are at rest. Easy inhales and exhales. This is a good place to start when you are practicing meditation. You can stay with easy breathing when you meditate, or deepen your inhales and exhales even further. There is no one absolute way to meditate; it is good to be aware of some options and of course to be aware of your breath.

Try it now: Sit comfortably and just notice your breath. Don't try to steer. Just be easy with it and yourself. If your attention wanders, just bring it back gently.

Long, Deep Breathing

This is the breathing you'll want to do when you're actively practicing yoga. When you take long deep inhales and exhales, your muscles can work efficiently and your mind can calm. Allow your movements to come out of your long, deep breath, and then everything you do with your body can flow with more ease. Try to avoid pushing or forcing your body. If you notice that you are pushing, your breath will probably shorten. When your breath shortens, simply guide it back.

Try it now: Sit up tall, sit comfortably. Close your eyes and begin to rest your attention on your breath. Lengthen and deepen your inhales and exhales, setting a full, deep, and even pace of breathing. Continue breathing at this pace for a few minutes. How do you feel?

Darth Vader Breath

Ujjayi breathing, dubbed Darth Vader breath because when you do it you sound like Darth Vader, focuses the mind during yoga and meditation practice and also specifically stimulates the vagus nerve, which sets off signals in the body that make you happy.

Try it now: Sit up tall, wherever you can sit comfortably. Close your eyes and begin to rest your attention on your breath. Lengthen and deepen your inhales and exhales, setting a nice, full, deep, and even pace of breathing. Constrict the back of your throat slightly so when you inhale and exhale you are making a soft hissing sound. Continue breathing this way for a few minutes. How do you feel? Any different from the exercise prior with just the long, deep breaths?

Alternate Nostril Breathing

Alternate nostril breathing calms the nervous system, eases anxiety, clears congestion and leaves you feeling pretty happy . . . even after just a few minutes of inhaling and exhaling. It's great to practice alternate nostril breathing every day, if only for a few moments. If you are headed into a meeting or an event that you are anxiously anticipating, do some alternate nostril breathing a few moments before to ease the stress. Alternate nostril breathing is also perfect to practice before meditation to center your body and focus the mind. When you have a cold, allergies, or any congestion, do it every day that you are experiencing these not-so-nice symptoms.

Try it now: Sit up tall, making sure you are also sitting comfortably. With your right hand, curl down your index and middle finger into your palm. You'll use your ring finger and your thumb, which is a perfect space for your nose to rest between. This hand position will help you alternate between nostrils as you inhale and exhale.

Press your ring finger over your left nostril and inhale for four counts through your right nostril. Close off your right nostril with your thumb so both sides of your nostrils are closed. Hold all the air in for four counts. Release your ring finger and let all the air out your left nostril for four counts. Reverse this pattern starting with inhaling through the left nostril, holding both closed, and exhaling out the right side. Repeat this breathing pattern for three to five minutes.

Bellows Breathing

Bellows breathing is great to clear out your entire system both physically and mentally. You'll take short and fast exhales through the nose, letting the inhales come naturally. Bellows breathing gives your circulatory and nervous systems a quick cleanse, along with a boost of energy.

Try it now: Sit up tall, and sit comfortably. Take a long and deep inhale. Exhale sharply through the nose, let the inhale follow naturally and repeat at a medium pace for a few seconds. If you feel comfortable start to pick up the pace until you are exhaling pretty rapidly. Try to continue for thirty seconds to a minute. When you are ready to finish, slow down your exhales gradually until you can resume normal, deep breathing.

Breath of Fire

If you are ever cold and need to get warmed up quickly, breath of fire is the technique for you. Breath of fire generates heat and increases your level of energy. After a few seconds of this breath you will feel rejuvenated and energized. Performing breath of fire oxygenates your blood, helping it detoxify and remove waste more effectively. It also balances the nervous system, massages the internal organs, and improves the digestive system.

Try it now: Sit up tall and straight, and sit comfortably. Take a long and deep inhale. Exhale all your air out. Begin to breathe rapidly in and out through the nose like really fast sniffing.

During those moments that we are resting our attention on the breath, we are removed from the way we experience time throughout the rest of the day. Time literally will seem to slow during meditation, and when you come out of these breathing meditations the amount of time that did or didn't go by may surprise you. Have you ever had an experience where time seemed to slow down greatly or even stand still? Athletes talk about this phenomenon as being "in the zone." After Michael Jordan scored thirty-five points in the first half of one game he said, "I can't explain it. It feels like time stands still. This bucket is huge, it's like I can't miss. I'm in the zone."

We all have the ability to get in this zone by cultivating a regular meditation practice. And the best part is it only gets better. The more you practice, the more zoned in you will be!

Why is this so important? Because of the domino effect that comes with such mindful attention to ourselves. Keep reading. Before we get to the cures, I'd like to securely connect a few more of these yoga dots into the whole that is a healthy life.

THE DOMINO EFFECT

With a regular yoga practice, we can manage stress as well as learn to let go of the things that build it in the first place. We can cleanse the body and mind on a regular basis. We can prevent so many ailments from ever becoming issues, and deal much better with ones that do.

The more we practice yoga and meditate the more we become sensitive to the foods that are good for us. A really transformative thing that happens very frequently when someone begins a regular yoga practice is that cravings actually shift from foods that weren't the healthiest to those that are nourishing and healing.

REAL-LIFE CURES: Leslie's Bacon-to-Broccoli Transformation

Leslie walked into the yoga studio and decided she was going to do yoga every day for two weeks. She had just been laid off and wanted to start a routine that made her feel good in her body and mind. Her eating habits weren't the best. At home she would snack on bacon in between meals, and at regular mealtimes eat a lot of fried and salty foods. She mentioned after just one week of yoga that her cravings had changed drastically. She noticed when she left class that she wanted to eat something fresh. She started making salads and greens for herself. She also felt an urge to prepare her own food, not grab it on the go while eating out every day, which was her habit pre-yoga. Leslie's bacon-to-broccoli transformation isn't so shockingly unique either. Practicing yoga draws your attention to how you feel and what you need to feel good. The body and mind want healthy fuel. We don't treat ourselves to what we actually need a lot of the time because we are so out of touch with what *we* actually want.

The more yoga we do the more we're drawn to other healthy practices. Not only will you naturally start to crave healthier foods, you'll want to treat yourself better, spend more quality time with friends and family, and even become more sensitized to life's daily wonders. All of that breathing and paying attention works wonders.

TIME TO MAKE THE YOGA: WHAT HABITS ARE HELPING/HURTING YOU?

You're going to need a piece of paper and something to write with for this exercise. Take a few moments to reflect on the age-old cures that you have adopted and made use of in your life. It can be a yoga practice, reading, a type of exercise or artistic activity, long walks with friends, or a fantastic tip that a close friend or family member passed down to you.

On one side of your paper list all of the healthy living practices and habits you integrate into your life that benefit you on a daily basis. It doesn't have to be anything super serious. It can be as simple as taking a hot bath to unwind at the end of a long week.

Now on the other side of the paper write down habits you have that aren't the best, ones you'd like to change in your life. The list could include items like unwinding from stress, eating fewer processed foods, and drinking less alcohol, or bigger issues like stopping smoking or finding alternatives to prescription drugs, if possible.

Now that you have your list, observe without judging which side is longer. Is it the healthy habits or the habits you'd like to change? Simply look at it without judging.

Now that you have your habits right there in front of you, it is time to get to work. If you have a lot of things listed on the healthy practices side, decide how you are going to keep them integrated into your life and add even more if possible. Be specific, like "I will meditate for ten minutes before I go to sleep tonight" or "I will cook a healthy dinner of broccoli and quinoa tonight." Think of ways to share your healthy habits with people close to you. We need to keep these positive behaviors alive by passing them to others.

Now if your list was heavy on the habits you'd like to change, that's okay too. We start where we are, and as I've said, we're always right where we need to be. So let's make a plan.

Starting right now, decide on one thing you would like to change. It doesn't have to be dramatic. It can be as simple as promising that for the rest of the day whenever you feel yourself getting stressed you will watch your breath for five long, deep breaths. Or maybe, for today, you will not eat any processed foods, and you try the same for tomorrow. Whatever your challenges are, decide to take one on today. Breathe new life into it and you'll transform it into something beautiful . . . just like you'll transform yourself.

ZENSPIRATION

Take a deep breath. The present moment is where everything is always happening and where you need to be. Each breath brings you right into the present.

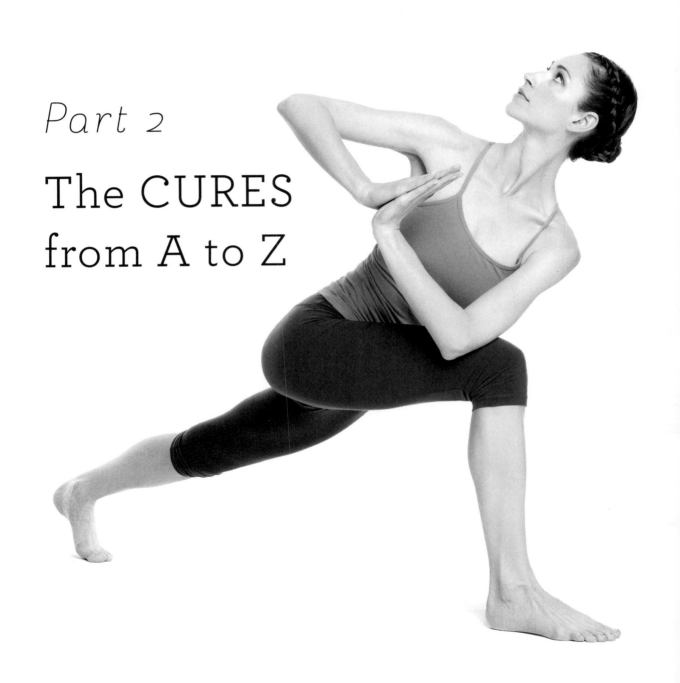

Part 2

The CURES
from A to Z

When we're already experiencing pain, careful attention is needed to navigate through it and begin to heal.

One great thing about yoga: its focus is on us, rather than simply on our problems. We are treating our entire selves, not an illness. When you cure with yoga, you are curing the root of whatever is in the way. It's not simply a matter of masking the problem without touching the cause, an approach that too often leads to more problems and side effects springing up elsewhere.

The yoga poses, movements, and breathing techniques are designed to heal your body, creating intricate patterns that correct imbalance in the nervous system on a cellular level. The poses are designed to regulate your thyroid, blood flow, digestive system, and even brain activity. Yoga helps you rebuild and reinvigorate yourself from the inside out. Who doesn't deserve that? Healthy and happy. It works for me … but that's because as I've said it before: Yoga cures.

Often the simplest of answers to a problem lies right in front of us. With yoga, it's even closer than that. It's right inside of us.

I love the universal nature of this quote from Henry Ford because it speaks to so many things, including the healing ability of yoga. Yoga has mostly to do with what is going on in your mind. If you believe something is possible, then it can be. If you believe something is impossible then it is for you, until you change your mind. And the kicker is no one can change your mind for you, but you.

Yoga teaches us to be at ease in our bodies and minds. If we can learn to be at ease, our nervous, muscular, circulatory, immune, and hormonal systems can operate beautifully and keep us radiantly healthy throughout our whole lives. On the other side of things, when our bodies and minds are tense, wound up, and stressed out, all sorts of things start to go haywire.

If you don't believe you can do it, it won't work. So I suggest you start believing in yourself. I will guide you in the direction of techniques that can work for you but you have to do the work all on your own. Believing in yourself is your best cure.

Anything is possible. Whether you think you can or you think you can't, you're right. —Henry Ford

TOOLS OF THE TRADE

A few things you might want to have handy to assist you while you practice:

2 yoga blocks: You can pick these up at most all-purpose stores, and of course online. Yoga blocks are great helpers for many poses. If you don't have yoga blocks, no worries, you can substitute with some firm pillows for most of the poses.

1 blanket: This can be any blanket that you don't mind lying on.

1 yoga mat: You will probably want a mat to practice on to provide some padding and help keep you from slipping. If you don't have a mat, you can still practice wherever you are—on the wood floor, a rug, or a carpet. Just go easy on the knees!

ONE MORE THING...

The following cures are aimed at inspiring you to ignite and maintain a lasting path of radiant health for your life. I hope they will alleviate pain, reduce stress, release tension, and promote health, happiness, well-being, and peace of mind in you.

These cures are not designed to be a quick fix or Band-Aid for a pressing issue, or substitution for other care and attention to your health and well-being. Please use your best judgment always when practicing yoga, and also when self-diagnosing symptoms.

For yoga to cure, you have to be present, honest with yourself, and in the moment. How you do the poses is what's important for healing, not just putting your body in the positions. By paying careful attention to your breath and to the rest of you, you'll be on your way to curing yourself from many of life's little problems and even some of the big ones. Even when a cure isn't possible, yoga can help us gain perspective and live our best life with whatever conditions we have.

Each cure in the book illustrates a few key yoga poses selected to have a specific effect, or a set of effects, on your body and mind. Whether aimed at alleviating allergies, acne, PMS, or hangovers, these cures are your springboard to fantastic health and happiness. Think of these cures as different entry points to a life filled with energy, vigor, and zest.

These cures will work if you have patience, ease of mind, ease of body, ease of breath, and, again, pay careful attention.

Please respect your body, go easy on yourself, and, of course, have fun. Yoga is supposed to be enjoyable. Enjoy your breath. Enjoy your body. Enjoy your connection to yourself. Now let's make some yoga!

DAILY YOGA

To reap the vast benefits of yoga it's important to practice daily. Whether you are experiencing an ailment that we'll aim to remedy, or you are working toward a personal goal, or you simply want to maintain your health and happiness, consistency is essential.

If you are new to yoga and overwhelmed by the thought of rolling out your yoga mat every day for eternity, begin with a very simple meditation each day instead. It only takes a moment to check in with the breath, and once you do, you'll probably get hooked. Regular practice will soon be as natural as waking up in the morning. Make the time for yourself. Your health and happiness is worth it. I promise, you won't regret it.

Warming Up

Before each routine, if you'd like to add a warm-up, I suggest spending a few minutes in seated meditation. Follow this by a few minutes of sun salutations, so you can get centered and connected with your breath and begin to wake up and feel your entire body. Each time you practice will feel different, so allow your body to back off and adjust accordingly, depending on how you feel.

Seated Meditation

Sit up nice and tall, however you can sit most comfortably. Relax your shoulders, so that they are away from your ears. Rest your palms on your thighs (face up or face down, whichever is most comfortable for you) and close your eyes. Start to rest your attention on your breath. Watch your inhales come and exhales go. Settle your mind in the space between. Begin to lengthen and deepen your inhales and exhales, setting a slow, easy pace of breathing. If a thought starts to enter your mind, simply observe it like a cloud passing by. Let the thought pass and come back to your breath. Continue observing your breath for three to five minutes. You can use a stopwatch if that's handy, or you could simply feel it out and see how much time has actually passed when you open your eyes. Either way is useful.

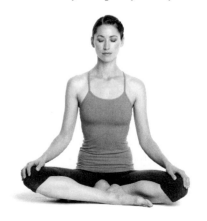

Sun Salutations

There are many different variations of sun salutations. This is a very simple version that is designed to open up your entire body. Move gently between each of these poses. Feel free to add in more or fewer movements depending on how you'd like to tailor your practice. Some of the poses you will be breathing through with either one deep inhale or one long exhale, and some of them you can hold for one to five full breaths, or longer if you prefer. The most important thing is to feel your way through the sequence, allow your body to move with ease, and enjoy the feeling of moving gently through space. Every inhale creates space and length in your body and mind. Every exhale releases tension and moves you into that new space. The deeper you breathe, the more you open up. So breathe fully and deeply and enjoy the ride!

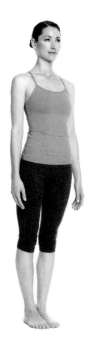

Standing

Stand at the top of your yoga mat. Feet are parallel and slightly apart, under your hip bones. Your hip bones aren't at the outside of your hips so make sure your feet aren't too far apart. You can check by placing two fists between your feet. That's about the width of your hipbones. Close your eyes and bring your attention to your breath. Lengthen and deepen your inhales and exhales and continue breathing at this nice slow pace for five full breaths. Gently open your eyes.

Standing Arm Reach

Inhale and lift your arms out to your sides and up, filling all the space with your breath and your movement. Relax your tailbone downward and lift your chest. Keep your shoulders relaxed and down and look up while keeping your face and your forehead relaxed.

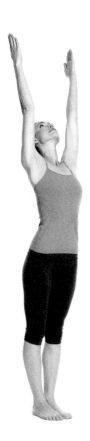

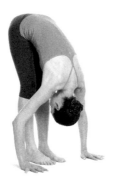

Standing Forward Bend

Exhale and bend your trunk forward over your legs. Let your head and neck relax and hang heavy. If your hamstrings feel tight keep a slight bend in your knees to give them some more space to relax and open. Press your fingertips on the ground.

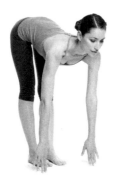

Standing Forward Bend with Arch

Inhale, look forward and lengthen out your back, so that it lifts up to horizontal. Let your fingertips graze the ground. If that's too much stress on your hamstrings, press your hands lightly into your shins to get a nice length in your spine.

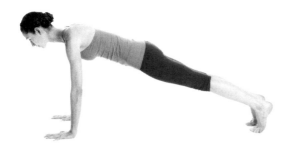

Plank

Bend your knees as much as you need to press your palms into the ground. Press into your hands and step your feet straight back, bringing your body into a straight line from the top of your head through your heels. Keep your stomach nice and strong and lift the front of your thighs up. Stay here for five long, deep breaths. If this is too intense, gently lower your knees to the floor.

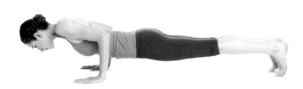

Plank Push-Up

You can either do this with your knees lifted, or lowered. Listen to your body. Bend your elbows straight back and lower your body halfway down in one straight line until your upper arms are parallel to the ground. If a half push-up is too intense simply lower slowly all the way down to your belly by bending your elbows straight back.

Up Dog

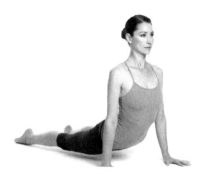

Lower your knees gently to the ground. If you did plank with your knees lowered, then they will be all set. Roll your shoulders down and lift your chest up through your arms with a big inhale. Straighten your arms as much as feels comfortable, while keeping your shoulders down. If you straighten your arms and your back feels pinched, bend the elbows and continue to lift your chest through your arms until you feel good. Don't be shy about adding a little movement if needed to keep the pose fresh and help open up your back. Sway your torso a bit from side to side if that feels good. Remember, keep your body easy, never forced or tense.

Child's Pose

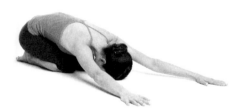

Move out of up dog so that you accordion your body and gently shift your hips to your heels. Arms should be long and rested in front of you along either side of your head. Rest your forehead on the ground and breathe deeply into your back. Stay here for five long, deep breaths. Observe the sensations in your body as they gently come and go, the same way you watched your thoughts go by like passing clouds earlier. Take three long, full deep breaths here.

Down Dog

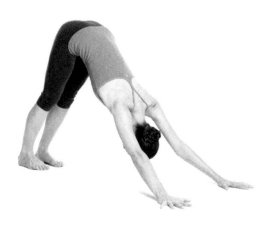

Spread your fingers wide, like you are digging into wet sand, lift your hips, tuck your toes and lift back into down dog. Reach your heels down toward the ground, relax your shoulders and neck. Keep some easy movements happening in the pose to encourage the body to open and prevent it from getting stuck in a static position. Gently sway from side to side. Stay in down dog for five long, deep breaths.

When you are ready, slowly walk your feet up to your hands and return to your standing forward bend. Roll up to standing, one vertebra at a time. Once you reach the top, inhale and lift your arms out and up, filling up all the space with all of you. As you exhale gently release your arms down by your sides. Repeat this simple sun salutation variation five times or more to create some heat in the body and ease of mind.

Aches and Pains

Aches and pains in our backs, necks, and joints can creep up on us over time or happen suddenly. However they arrive, they can be a huge burden and limitation on our mobility, increase our stress levels, and disrupt our peace of mind. The best way to cure aches and pains is to prevent them from finding us in the first place. A regular yoga and meditation practice can help a lot with that, especially the simple yoga and breathing techniques that follow.

In a study conducted by Dr. Fadel Zeidan at Wake Forest University in North Carolina, fifteen volunteers who had no previous meditation experience took four twenty-minute classes in a type of meditation called focused attention. After the training, a small area of skin on each patient's right leg was heated to a pain-inducing level for five minutes, while an MRI monitored pain signals in the brain. Dr. Zeidan said, "We found a big effect—about 40 percent reduction in pain intensity and a 57 percent reduction in pain unpleasantness. Meditation produced a greater reduction in pain than even morphine or other pain-relieving drugs, which typically reduce ratings by about 25 percent."

So now we know that meditation can alter our mental perception of painful experiences, which is pretty useful. We can also utilize physical yoga (moving meditation) to harness our ability to change the state of our bodies. Taking both into account we can send our aches and pains on their way for good!

REAL-LIFE CURES: Tara Lets the Pain Roll off Her Shoulders

I have to confess I've had my share of aches and pains. One I should have been able to prevent is an intense pain that found its way from my shoulder into my upper and lower back from always carrying a way-too-heavy purse on my right shoulder. Not good! I know it's hard to remember to switch shoulders, but trust me, it's worth it if you carry a heavy bag. Or, better yet, get a backpack! When this sharp and lasting pain took hold, I put myself on a regimen of gentle, supported, back-opening yoga. It took several days to work itself out, but it finally did. So now I hold my bag in my hand and switch hands every so often to even things out.

THE ACHES AND PAINS YOGA CURE

"Aches and pains" is a pretty broad category to cover in one entry, but the yoga fundamentals in dealing with most pain are going slow, breathing deeply, and, you guessed it, paying attention. When you move very slowly, you're giving your body a chance to communicate with you about where you are misaligned by telling you if what you are doing is helping or creating more pain. With yoga, if something is painful, always back out of it slowly and come to a neutral position so you can recover fully. Allow any uncomfortable sensations to leave your body before you move on. The age-old advice "take it easy" applies when working with our aches and pains.

Try this routine whenever you are experiencing mild aches and pains. Approach it with care and ease. Again, make sure to back off from anything that causes more pain. A good sign that pain is building in your system is face scrunching and shortness of breath. If you feel either, dial it back. Allow yourself the time and space for the body to heal and the mind to settle.

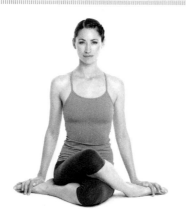

Cow Face

Start kneeling with your hands on the ground for support. Bring your right leg in front of your left leg so that your knees are directly in a line. Move your feet out to the sides. Gently sit your hips back until they reach the floor. Your knees will now be stacked on top of each other. If there is tension in the knees or hips, place a pillow or a block under your hips to allow more room for the hips and knees to open without stress. Lift your chest so that the muscles feel open and your shoulders are back, and sit up tall. Stay here for ten long, deep breaths.

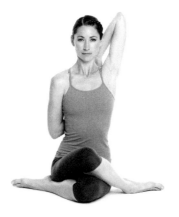

Cow Face with Shoulder Opener

If you have a greater range of motion, inhale and raise your left arm straight up. Bend your elbow and let your hand relax on your back. Bend your right elbow and reaching behind your back, stretch your right hand up toward your left hand. If the hands meet link them. If not, don't worry about it. You're getting a nice opening in the shoulders either way. Spread your fingers wide and open your elbows a little further. Stay here for ten long, deep breaths. Make sure to do the other side too.

Supported Bridge with 2 Blocks

Grab two yoga blocks. Place one flat on the ground vertically, so if you were to lie down it would be along your spine. Sit a few inches in front of the block. Recline on the block so that it is supporting your middle and upper back. Take your other block and place it under your head. It should be very comfortable, so shift yourself around as much as needed until this position feels really good.

Once you are settled take a few long inhales through the nose and exhales through the mouth. Continue with natural, long, deep breaths and stay here for as long as it feels comfortable. To come out of it, roll off the blocks and onto your right side. Take a few breaths here to recover.

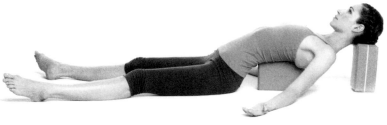

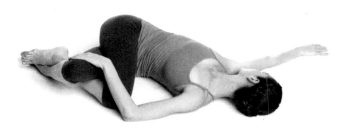

Reclining Eagle Twist

Lie down on your back. Take a big inhale in through your nose, and a long exhale out through your mouth. Relax and breathe naturally for a few moments to allow your body to settle and your mind to calm.

When you are ready, bend your knees and plant your feet on the ground next to your hips. Lift your hips, move them toward your right side and lower them down. Cross your right leg over your left leg. Hug your knees into your chest and relax them over toward your left side. Extend your right arm out to your right side and look toward your hand. Rest your left hand on your left knee to encourage the knees to relax toward the ground. Stay here for twenty long, deep breaths. When you are ready, bring your legs back to the center and try the other side, too.

Squat with Neck Release

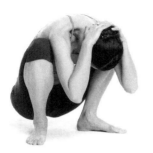

Stand up tall. Scoot your feet open until they are about shoulder distance apart. Turn your feet slightly outward and your heels in. Bend your knees and lower your hips toward the ground. Your heels should be firmly on the ground. If your heels don't meet the ground easily, you can place a blanket under them to bring the floor to you and create more stability in the pose. Stay here for five long, deep breaths.

Interlace your hands gently at the base of your neck. Relax your head and neck forward and allow your back to round. Don't pull your head down, but hold firmly and steadily at the neck to encourage your neck to release. Stay here for five long, deep breaths. To come out of the pose, place your fingertips on the ground behind your tailbone, and sit down easily.

Reclined Butterfly Spine Opener (with blanket)

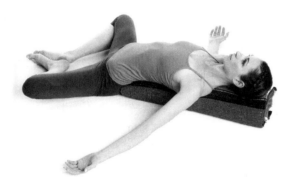

Roll up a blanket lengthwise. For extra height, roll two blankets together. Sit up and place the blanket behind you next to your tailbone. Gently roll down so your spine rests along the blanket. Bring the bottoms of your feet together. Relax your arms out to your sides. Close your eyes and rest here for twenty long, deep breaths.

Acne

For some of us, acne was part of the growing pains of our teenage years; others battle with acne in their adult lives. Both can cause stress, which leads to more and worse breakouts. We know from experience that yoga reduces stress, and we know that a lot of people who practice yoga regularly have that "yoga glow" (their skin is dewy and fresh looking). Ever wonder how some people get their glow? It's not from expensive creams, Botox, or surgeries. Just yoga . . . and all the healthy activities a regular yoga practice naturally points you toward.

Acne forms when glands in the follicles of your skin produce sebum, an oil that lubricates your skin. When the sebum makes its way to the surface of your skin, it carries along dead skin cells. When the mixture clogs a pore, bacteria horn in, leading to inflammation and acne. Yoga comes to the rescue because of acne's connection to stress. The hormone that goes along with the feeling of stress is cortisol. When you experience stress, your adrenal glands release it, which triggers a bunch of things to happen in your body, including an increased production of sebum. Too much sebum means clogged pores and acne. Now you know one more reason why you should reduce stress; looking good is a great benefit, feeling less stressed is priceless.

THE ACNE YOGA CURE

Heightened stress levels make all sorts of not-so-good things happen chemically in our bodies. These stress triggers can set us up for sickness and eventually turn into disease. Acne is a relatively benign outcome of stress and there is no harm in trying yoga as a cure, as it's widely accepted that a regular yoga practice will reduce your stress levels.

Try this routine as often as you'd like. Three times a week is a great start! It is designed to put you in a few simple positions that require your muscles to work for you, while challenging your mind to be calm. If you can be comfortable during a plank pose, for instance, you will find ease in most other circumstances in your life. So plank up and look forward to a more acne-free and stress-free life.

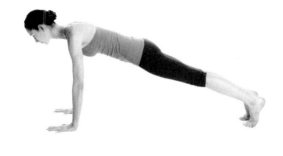

Plank

Get on all fours. Make sure your wrists are under your shoulders and your knees are under your hips. Spread your fingers wide, like you are digging into some nice, wet sand. Tuck your toes under and straighten your legs and arms, bringing your body into a straight line from the top of your head through the bottoms of your heels. Keep your stomach nice and strong and lift the front of your thighs up. Stay here for five, long, deep breaths. If this is too intense gently lower your knees to the floor. Always make sure you can breathe easily during this pose.

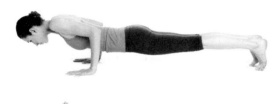

Plank Push-Up

You can do this with either your knees lifted, or lowered for a bit less challenging version. Listen to your body and adjust accordingly. Bend your elbows back and lower your body in one straight line half way down until your upper arms are parallel to the ground. Keeping your body in a straight line, press back up.

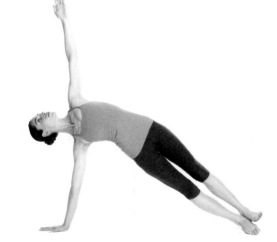

Side Plank

From your plank pose press into your right hand, lift your hips slightly, and roll to the outside edge of your right foot. Lengthen your left arm out so that it's straight and in line with your shoulders. Look up at your left hand. You can either keep the feet as they are, stack them on top of each other if you feel steady, or if this is too much, lower your right knee down so you can feel more stable. Stay here for two long, deep inhales and exhales. Roll down and through a plank pose and try the other side.

Bow

From a plank, bend your elbows and slowly lower down until you are lying on your belly. Bend your knees, and reaching back and around, grab the outside of your ankles with your hands. Gently press your feet into your hands. Your body will lift and your back will arch. Don't force your back to open, but use the pressure of your feet in your hands to take your body to where it can move easily with your breath. Stay here for three long, deep breaths and slowly lower down. If grabbing both feet at once isn't possible try doing one at a time.

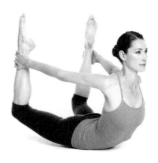

ADD/ADHD

For many children and adults, a wandering mind is more than a distracting problem. It is the core symptom of ADD and ADHD. Yoga has been shown to help focus and calm the mind and ease the problems of people suffering from these disorders. Even if you don't suffer from either one, as a society we are constantly "on," constantly overstimulated. We're plugged into our mobile devices and constantly sending and receiving messages all day long. It can be easy to get caught up in this frenzy and hard to step back and focus on one thing at a time. The time we spend on the computer can further shorten our attention span.

A study randomly selected children with ADHD to either practice yoga or follow a more traditional exercise routine. Hands down, the winner was clear. The children who practiced yoga improved their attention and had fewer ADHD symptoms versus the exercise group.

THE ADD AND ADHD YOGA CURE

Just as stress reduction has a deeper effect on your overall health, cultivating the ability to pay attention takes you much further than only improving your ability to focus. Paying attention without getting involved in our racing thoughts and responding to every impulse of our bodies without consideration is essential in developing lasting ease of body and mind. Living with a body and mind that are at ease is much more enjoyable than living with a mind that shoots from thought to thought like a ping pong ball, fidgeting and twitching to work out its restlessness.

This routine is designed to relax and focus the mind through a bit of physical effort. Most of us have experienced a super hard and long day, the kind where, at its end, all you want to do is go home, lie down on the couch, and veg out for the night. As adults we find ourselves polarized between effort and relaxation. Either we are working really hard and simultaneously building stress and tension in our bodies and minds, or relaxing like pros. If we can learn to find the ease in our effort, we can actually be relaxing all of the time.

When we find this ease in our lives, our minds can drop all the excess activity that isn't useful and just clogs up our brains and bodies like a backed-up drain. Think of this routine as Drano for a restless mind. Try it every day and set up a great new habit.

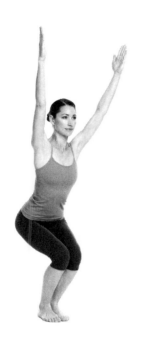

Chair

Stand up tall with your feet parallel to each other, under your hipbones. Shoulders should be in a line with your hips. Stand with your eyes closed for three long, deep breaths. On your next inhale, bend your knees and sink your hips down like you are sitting in a chair. Reach your arms up toward your ears, keeping your shoulders blades down your back. Relax your face. Allow your muscles to work for you without getting involved. If thoughts begin to enter your mind, observe them and then gently send them on their way. Stay here for five long, deep breaths. If your body starts to feel like it's working to stay in this position, that's a good thing, it just means you are alive and have a functioning body. Breathe fuller and deeper to give your body what it needs here.

Standing Forward Bend Shoulder Opener

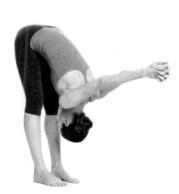

Stand comfortably with your feet a few inches apart. Inhale deeply. As you exhale, gently fold your torso forward over your legs. Interlace your hands behind you and let your arms fall over your back. If your hamstrings feel tense, bend your knees slightly and rest your belly on your thighs. Relax more deeply into the pose with each exhale. Begin to lengthen your exhales a bit more than your inhales; this will encourage the body to open and the mind to settle. Stay here for five long, deep breaths.

Standing

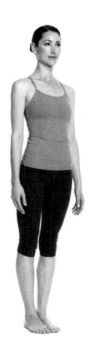

From the shoulder opener pose, release your clasped hands and rest your fingertips on the floor. Bend your knees slightly, relax your head and neck, and slowly roll up to a standing position, one vertebra at a time. Your shoulders should be aligned above your hips and the top of your head should feel almost like it's floating up. Take a long deep inhale through your nose and exhale out through your mouth. Close your eyes and bring your attention to your breath. Lengthen and deepen your inhales and exhales and continue breathing at this nice slow pace for five full breaths. Gently open your eyes.

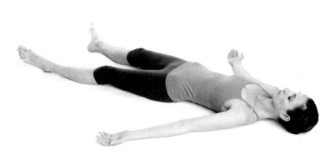

Corpse

Lie down on your back. Open your legs hip width apart, or a bit wider, depending on what's most comfortable for you. Relax your arms a bit out to your sides, palms facing up. Take a big inhale through your nose, exhale all the air out through your mouth. Repeat the same breathing pattern twice more. Now let your breathing be natural and simply relax for three to five minutes.

When you are ready to come out of the pose, slowly start to deepen your breath. Roll your wrists and ankles. Gently hug your knees into your chest and rock up to sitting.

INHALE/HOLD, EXHALE/HOLD

Giving your mind a specific task to do is often a very effective way to calm and focus a restless mind. We're going to practice a simple breathing pattern, creating a meditation aimed at calming and focusing your mind.

Inhale slowly through your nose as you count to four, one being the beginning of your inhale and four being at the very top. At the top hold all the air in for another count to four, and then release the air slowly for another slow count of four. Hold without breathing for another slow count of four. Begin the cycle again with your next inhale and repeat this breathing pattern ten times.

If you'd like to continue on with this meditation for a while longer after you have completed your breathing pattern, return to natural, easy inhales and exhales. If your mind begins to wander, gently guide it back to the breath. If you feel restless always feel free to adjust your seated position. Continue meditating for as long as you'd like. Try to keep this up every day for a week as a first goal. From there, hopefully, you'll be hooked on the great benefits and you'll continue doing it permanently. Enjoy!

Allergies

Whether they are seasonal or affect you year-round, if you suffer from allergies, it's no fun. Runny nose, sneezing, stuffy head, loss of sleep, and fuzzy concentration are symptoms that can be reduced and often done away with entirely by a regular yoga practice and some specific breathing techniques. Allergies are worsened by stress, which causes physiological responses that include the release of stress hormones and histamine, and triggers inflammation. "Relaxation diminishes the fight-or-flight response and thereby reduces allergic symptoms," says Jeff Migdow, MD, director of Prana yoga teacher training at the Open Center in New York as well as a holistic physician at the Kripalu Center for Yoga and Health in Lenox, Massachusetts.

THE ALLERGY YOGA CURE

In curing allergies with yoga, we need to calm the nervous system so the body can begin to work properly again. We can use our yoga practice as a tool to see if we push and force our breath and bodies and cause aggravation to our systems, or if we are very calm and easy while we live/practice. Calm and easy is the goal. There are no extra points in yoga for clenching up and muscling your way through.

This routine is designed to calm the nervous system, open the lungs, and strengthen immunity; the three together can help alleviate allergy symptoms. It's useful to practice these techniques regularly even when not experiencing allergy symptoms so you can continue to shore up your immunity and improve your overall health and well-being. The best cure is always prevention. Do this routine daily when you are experiencing allergy symptoms, and three times a week when you are not.

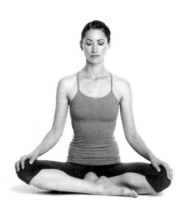

Bellows Breathing

Begin with seated mediation. After a few minutes of meditation you'll be ready to begin bellows breathing, which increases oxygen and decreases carbon dioxide in the blood, cleanses the body's systems, and clears the mind.

Make sure you remain in a comfortable seated position. This technique can be pretty intense so you want to make sure you're not standing.

You'll take short and fast exhales through the nose. Your inhales will follow the exhales naturally, but don't force the inhales. Start slow and work to building the breathing to a quicker rate.

Take a long, deep inhale. Exhale sharply through the nose, let the inhale follow naturally and repeat at a medium pace for a few seconds. If you feel comfortable, start to pick up the pace until you are exhaling pretty rapidly. Try to continue for thirty seconds to a minute. When you are ready to finish, slow down your exhales gradually until you can resume normal, deep breathing.

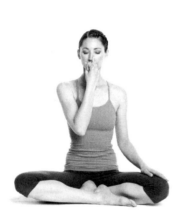

Alternate Nostril Breathing

This breathing technique has some wonderful benefits, including soothing the nervous system, cleansing the lungs, calming the mind, and enhancing rest and relaxation.

Staying seated, curl the index and middle fingers of your right hand, so that they touch the insides of your palm. For this exercise, you'll use your ring finger and your thumb, which provide a perfect space for your nose to rest between.

Press your ring finger over your left nostril and inhale for four counts through your right nostril. Close off your right nostril with your thumb so both nostrils are closed. Hold the air in for four counts. Release your ring finger and exhale the air out through your left nostril for four counts. Reverse this pattern starting with inhaling through the left nostril, holding both closed, and exhaling out the right side. Repeat this breathing pattern for three to five minutes.

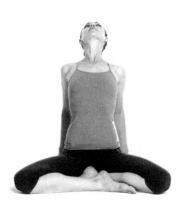

Seated Chest Lift

From your comfortable, seated position move your arms back behind you and press your fingertips into the ground alongside your hips. Inhale and gently lift your chest straight up. Feel your spine lengthening. If it feels easy, lift your hips up to create even more length in the chest and spine. Lower your hips down gently as you exhale. Repeat this movement twice more.

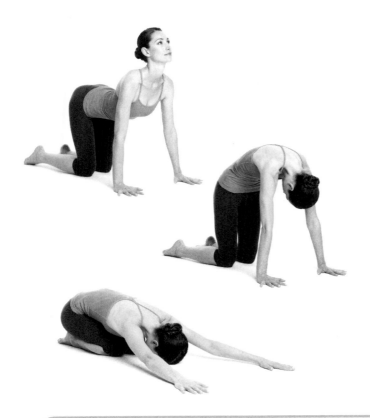

Cat/Cow

From seated chest lift, come onto all fours with your wrists directly under your shoulders and your knees directly under your hips. Spread your fingers wide, like you are digging into wet sand. Bring your spine to a neutral position and take a few long, deep breaths. As you inhale, drop your belly down toward the ground, allow your back to arch, and look up into a cow pose. As you exhale, round your back like a cat and look inward. Repeat this movement several times, moving along with your breath. Try to avoid pushing your body to achieve a shape, but rather breathe deeply and allow your body to open up to where your breath can take you right now.

Child's Pose

Gently come onto all fours. Relax your hips and sit back on your heels. Rest your forehead on the ground and breathe deeply into your back. Stay here for five long, deep breaths.

REAL-LIFE CURES: Justin's Fight with Flowers

I was sitting in a waiting room one spring day in Manhattan and a young man named Justin was sitting at reception and sneezing up a storm. There was a beautiful bouquet of fresh flowers sitting next to him on his desk. He looked at me and said nothing was working. He said he was taking all of the over-the-counter drugs for allergies, and every day his symptoms kept getting worse. The flowers were setting them off at that moment, but he said it was pretty bad all day long no matter what. I suggested moving the flowers to the waiting room table, and he thought that was a great idea. I picked them up and moved them. He said his thinking was even a little clouded and he felt just awful. I asked him if he was interested in learning a breathing technique that I thought could help him. He said he would try anything. I talked him through some alternate nostril breathing and we practiced it together for about two minutes. He said he felt a lot better from just the two minutes and would continue practicing on his work breaks and at home. If two minutes can help, imagine what a daily practice can do.

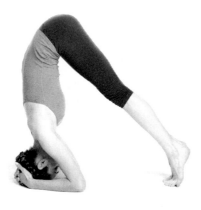

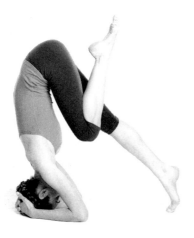

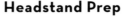

Headstand Prep

Headstands are great fun and they're great for you. They calm the brain, relieve stress, stimulate the pituitary and pineal glands, and strengthen the lungs, and are therapeutic for asthma and sinusitis. How to get ready for one?

Interlace your fingers loosely and place the sides of your hands on the floor. Place the top of your head in the space formed by your cupped hands. Stay here for a few breaths to get comfortable. If this is not comfortable, back out of it and go back to child's pose. Tuck your toes, straighten your legs, and lift your hips toward the sky. In this position you are getting a lot of the benefits of a headstand without your feet ever leaving the ground. Stay here for ten long, deep breaths and when you are ready, gently lower your knees to the ground and relax into child's pose.

Headstand

Mastering a headstand usually takes time, so remember to have patience and also to have fun.

If you are comfortable in the headstand prep position, start to walk your feet in toward your body so that your hips line up over your shoulders and your back is straight. Stay here for a few breaths. If you feel good, bend one knee in, bringing your heel to your hip. Bring it back down and try the other leg. If you are steady with one leg, try both legs at the same time. When your heels are pulled in toward your hips and you feel sturdy and stable, slowly extend your legs straight up. Stay for twenty long, deep breaths. When you are ready to come down, slowly lower one leg at a time and rest in child's pose for a few breaths.

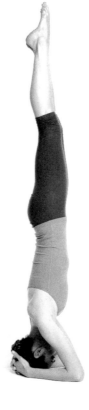

Anxiety

We all experience some anxiety from time to time. Whether we are stressed about an upcoming event or deadline, the outcome of a test, or in anticipation of an important meeting, how we deal with the feelings surrounding these moments is important. Stress is a part of life and doesn't necessarily disappear the moment we begin a regular yoga practice. But we do learn how to handle it a whole lot better. Yoga gives us physical and mental space between ourselves and a potential stressful situation.

In a German study published in 2005, twenty-four women who described themselves as "emotionally distressed" took two ninety-minute yoga classes a week for three months. A control group maintained normal activities and was asked not to begin a stress-reduction program during this time. At the end of the three months, women in the yoga group reported improvements in perceived stress, depression, anxiety, energy, fatigue, and well-being. Their depression scores improved by 50 percent, anxiety scores by 30 percent, and overall well-being by 65 percent. The control group reported no improvement.

THE ANXIETY YOGA CURE

Whether the stresses of daily life are a little or a lot overwhelming, yoga can help ease anxiety big-time and lead you back to feeling great again.

This routine is designed to ease excess tension in the body and mind. Do it daily to ease anxiety and calm the mind.

REAL-LIFE CURES: Tyler's Anxiety Disorder

Tyler started yoga for exercise. He soon found that after a few classes the yoga helped him relax and deal with feelings of overwhelming anxiety that he experienced on a daily basis. Tyler soon learned yoga is very different from other forms of exercise that he'd been involved with, like gym training and running. He found that when he moved his body with the direction of his breath instead of willing his mind to push his muscles, he experienced a profound sense of ease in his own skin. He was able to cultivate a lasting ability to relax and be easy in his body and mind through a regular practice.

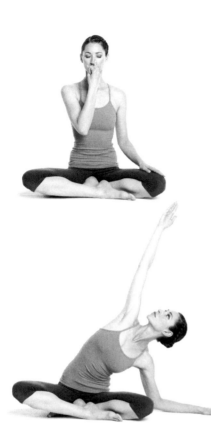

Alternate Nostril Breathing

Begin with a few moments of seated meditation. Staying seated, curl the index and middle fingers of your right hand, so that they touch the insides of your palm.

Press your ring finger over your left nostril and inhale for four counts through your right nostril. Close off your right nostril with your thumb so both nostrils are closed. Hold the air in for four counts. Release your ring finger and exhale the air out through your left nostril for four counts. Reverse this pattern starting with inhaling through the left nostril, holding both closed, and exhaling out the right side. Repeat this breathing pattern for three to five minutes.

Seated Easy Side Bend

Staying seated, gently lean over toward your left side and press your left palm and forearm into the ground alongside your body. Extend your right arm straight up overhead. Stay here for three long, deep breaths then try the other side.

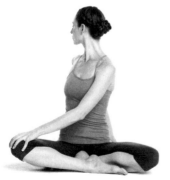

Seated Easy Twist

Staying seated, inhale and lift your left arm straight up. As you exhale, grab your right knee with your left hand. Press your right fingertips into the ground behind your hips. Inhale and sit up tall. Exhale and twist your torso further toward the right.

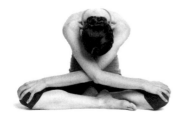

Seated Arm Cross, Hold Knees

From your seated twist keep your left hand on your right knee, inhale and lift your right arm up and over to grab hold of your left knee. Your hands should now be holding opposite knees. Relax your torso forward over your legs. Relax your head and neck. Stay here for three long, deep breaths then slowly roll up to sitting. Perform the same movements beginning with seated easy twist on the other side.

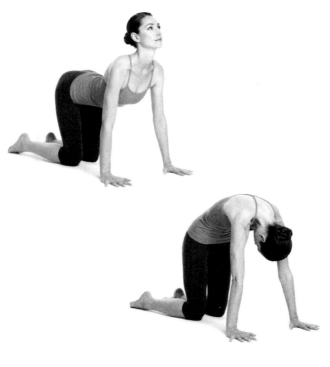

Cat/Cow

Come onto all fours, with your wrists directly under your shoulders and knees directly under your hips. Spread your fingers wide like you are digging into wet sand. Bring your spine to a neutral position and take a few long, deep breaths here. As you inhale, drop your belly down toward the ground, allow your back to arch and look up into a cow pose. As you exhale, round your back like a cat and look inward. Repeat this movement several times as you breathe. Try to avoid pushing your body to achieve a shape, but rather breathe deeply and allow your body to open up to where your breath can take you right now.

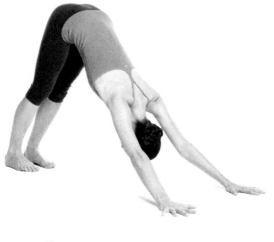

Down Dog

At the top of your next inhale in your cow pose, with your back arched and your gaze upward, tuck your toes, lift your hips, and press back to a down dog. Reach your heels toward the ground. Relax your shoulders and relax your head and neck. Stay here for five long, deep breaths.

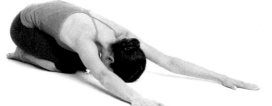

Child's Pose

From down dog, gently lower your knees to the ground, shift your hips back to sit on your heels, and relax your forehead on the ground. Stay here for five long, deep breaths.

Arthritis

If you have arthritis, practicing yoga can help in relieving joint pain, swelling, stiffness, and limited range of motion. A recent study conducted in the United Arab Emirates examined forty-seven rheumatoid arthritis patients who completed twelve sessions of Raj yoga (a gentle form of yoga). The study's author, Dr. Humeira Badsha, said, "While our study has been conducted in a small group of patients, the results show clear benefits for patients who regularly practice. We believe that practicing yoga for a longer term could in fact result in further significant improvements and we hope our study drives further research into the benefits of yoga in rheumatoid arthritis."

Meditation has also been shown to help people deal with arthritis. "Meditation is becoming increasingly popular as a way to treat chronic illness such as the pain caused by arthritis," said Dr. Christopher Brown, who conducted a meditation study on arthritis sufferers. "The results of the study confirm how we suspected meditation might affect the brain. Meditation trains the brain to be more present-focused and therefore to spend less time anticipating future negative events. This may be why meditation is effective at reducing the recurrence of depression, which makes chronic pain considerably worse."

THE ARTHRITIS YOGA CURE

To ease arthritis, practice meditation at least once per day for five to ten minutes. Work up to meditating twice per day, right when you wake up and before bed, for better results.

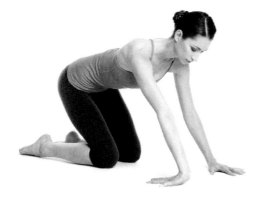

Hands and Knees Wrist Release

Come onto all fours. Make sure your wrists are directly under your shoulders, same for your knees and hips. Spread your fingers wide. Turn your right hand as far to the right as it will go, so the heel of your hand is facing forward and your fingers are facing your body. Press your palm into the ground. Gently put weight on the wrist and roll into the hand, breathing deeply into any tight areas that you find. Stay here for five long, deep breaths, then do the same with the other hand.

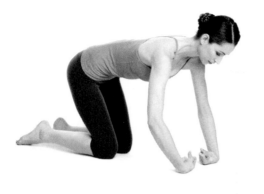

Hands and Knees Fist Release

Staying on all fours, make tight fists with both hands, bend your elbows out to the sides, and place the tops of your hands on the ground, your knuckles should be facing each other. Begin to straighten your elbows but only straighten as much as you can while keeping a tight fist. You should feel a stretch on the tops of your wrists.

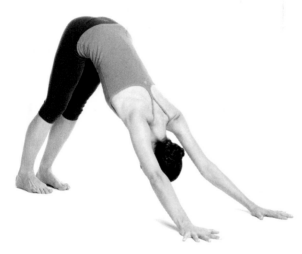

Down Dog

From all fours, tuck your toes, lift your hips, and press back into down dog. Reach your heels toward the ground. Relax your shoulders toward the ground and relax your head and neck. Stay here for five long, deep breaths.

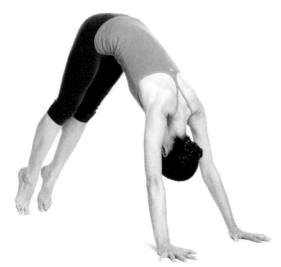

Down Dog, Lift Heels

In your down dog, inhale and lift high onto your toes, reaching your heels and hips straight up. Exhale and lower back into your down dog. Repeat twice more.

Bingeing

In a study published in 2009 by researchers in Australia, a group of women between the ages of twenty-five and sixty-three who were diagnosed with binge-eating disorder participated in a twelve-week yoga program aimed at reducing the severity of their disordered eating patterns. The group that practiced yoga reported significant reductions in their binge eating behaviors. The control group reported no significant change.

THE BINGEING YOGA CURE

The yoga cure when it comes to binge eating and other eating disorders often deals with settling the mind and curing it of anxiety, worry, fears, and the need for control. Yoga has a way of evening us out, and bringing us back to balance. When we have a hard time getting out of our own way, yoga is there to help.

This routine is designed to ease the mind and engage the body in a relaxed way. Do this routine daily.

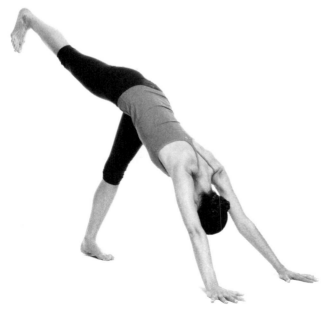

Down Dog Split

From your meditation, come onto all fours. Tuck your toes, lift your hips, and press your legs back into down dog. Inhale and lift your right leg straight up. Keep your hips square so the toes of your right foot are pointing down toward the ground. Lift up from the very back of your upper thigh. Press down firmly through both hands evenly. Reach out through both heels evenly.

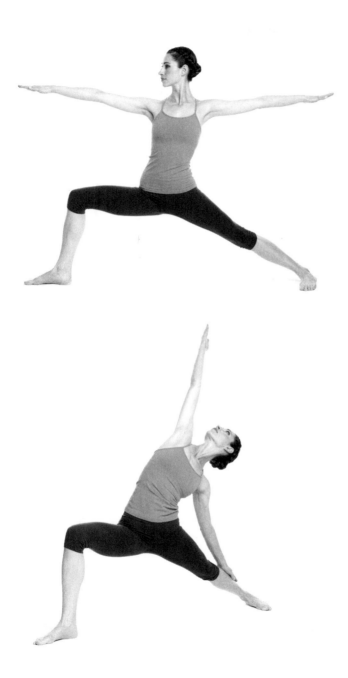

Warrior 2

Lift your right knee in toward your forehead and gently place your foot between your hands. Make sure your left heel is grounded, so that both feet are firmly planted on the ground. Press through your feet to standing, and bring your torso up in alignment over your hips. Angle your back foot so your toes are pointing slightly forward and your heel extends farther behind you. Open your arms straight out and away from your torso, right arm in front of you, and left arm behind you, palms down. Look over your front hand. Bend your right knee so your thigh is parallel to the ground. Stay here for ten long, deep breaths.

Reverse Warrior

Keeping your legs where they are, lean back toward your left leg, letting your left hand drape down toward your calf. Extend your right arm straight up overhead. Stay here for two long, deep breaths.

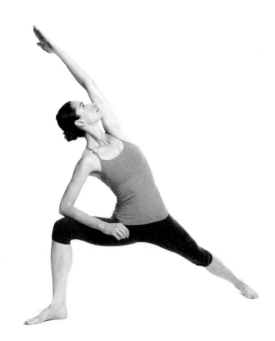

Extended Angle

Keeping your legs where they are, bring your torso forward over your front thigh. Press your right forearm into your right thigh and open your chest outward and up. Extend your left arm up and over your left ear. Look toward your left palm. Stay here for five long, deep breaths.

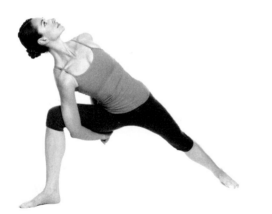

Extended Angle Bind

From your extended angle, if there is room, wrap your right arm under your upper thigh. Wrap your left arm around your back and hook your hands together. Lengthen your torso upward. Feel as if you are reaching upward with the top of your head and back through the outside edge of your back foot.

Come back into a down dog and do the routine on your other side.

Blurred Vision

A lot of us spend long hours in front of a computer screen, which can cause dry eye, eyestrain, and blurred or double vision. A recent study published in *Head & Face Medicine* reported the effects of eye yoga treatment on professional computer users in Bangalore, India. Employees of a software company either practiced yoga or took part in recreational activities daily for sixty days. The researchers found that the yoga group had a 30 percent decrease in eye problems, including dry eye and eyestrain. However, the recreational group had an increase in eye complaints.

THE BLURRED VISION YOGA CURE

If we spend a lot of our day at the computer, it's important to combat the eyestrain with yoga. There are several techniques that can soothe and repair vision. It's also a good idea to keep recreational computer time to a minimum to avoid further eye damage.

This routine is designed to ease stress on the eyes, improve relaxation of the muscles around the eyes, and improve vision. Do it daily to improve vision.

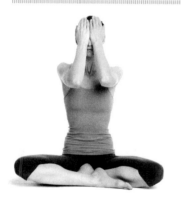

Calm Eyes

Sit comfortably. Relax your shoulders and sit up straight. Rub the palms of your hands together to get some heat going. Close your eyes, press the heels of your hands gently into your eye sockets, and rest your fingers against your forehead. Breathe naturally. Release your hands and let them hang at your sides.

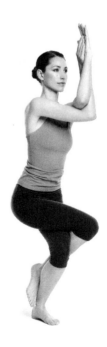

Eagle

Stand up and bring your feet parallel to each other, directly under your hips. Inhale and bend your knees, sitting back into a chair pose. Shift your weight onto your left leg and cross your right leg on top of your left leg, and hook your right foot around your ankle. Wrap your right arm under your left arm and bring your arms in front of your face. To stay balanced sit down through your hips as much as you lengthen up through your arms. Keep your gaze forward, through your arms. This pose strengthens your peripheral vision. Stay here for three long, deep breaths then try the other side.

Broken Heart

When your heart has been broken the last thing you might feel like doing is getting up and moving, but it can be the best thing for you. The clinical term "stress cardiomyopathy," known as "broken heart syndrome," can cause symptoms that mimic a heart attack. They typically occur after the death of a loved one, or a big physical strain like surgery, and the triggers are subtle and hard for doctors to pinpoint. A recent study published in the *Journal of the American Medical Association* has shown how different "broken heart syndrome" is from other heart conditions. Unlike a heart attack, where heart cells die, leaving scar tissue behind, with stress cardiomyopathy, the heart cells are temporarily stunned, but not irreversibly damaged. "This definitely shows, using MRI, that the pathophysiology of this condition is very different. It clearly separates this from other kinds of heart and muscle disorders," says Dr. Ilan S. Wittstein, a cardiologist and assistant professor at the Johns Hopkins University School of Medicine in Baltimore.

Yoga brings us back to our center, grounds us. When we are going through times that shake us to our core, troubling us emotionally, some gentle yoga poses can help us begin to heal. If you have a serious heart condition, of course, consult your doctor.

When we feel tender emotionally we can actually take advantage of the openness to take a look at how we feel about our life in general; we can use these hurts to gain some perspective. This perspective will help us grow and feel stable and get back to our usual happy selves.

THE BROKEN HEART YOGA CURE

The yoga cure for a broken heart is to simply get back on your feet and do some yoga, one breath at a time. It's the first step in getting back to feeling like yourself again.

This routine is designed to open the chest (heart area), get your body moving so you can get out of your head, and release tension, whether physical, emotional, or both, that is stored in your body. Try this routine whenever you have a broken heart. Do it daily until you start to feel like yourself again.

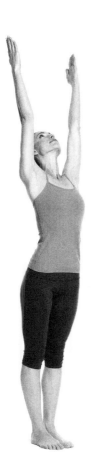

Standing Arm Reach

Stand tall with your feet a few inches apart, parallel to each other. Your arms should be loose, at your sides. Rest your shoulders down, and widen the area across your collarbones. Take a big, deep inhale and lift your arms up straight, as if you are embracing the sky. Drop your tailbone toward the ground and lift your chest up. As you exhale, lower your arms down to your sides. Repeat this twice more.

Low Lunge, Back Knee Down Arch

Come into a low lunge with your right leg forward and your left leg back. Sink your hips low toward the ground. Take three long, deep breaths here. Gently lower your back knee to the floor. Walk your fingertips back so they are under your shoulders. Sink your hips forward, drop your tailbone down, and arch your chest up. Stay here for five long, deep breaths.

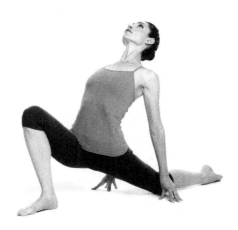

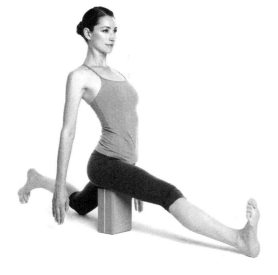

Split (with block)

Grab a block. From your low lunge, lower your back knee down to the ground. Flex your front foot and slide your heel out in front of you. Place the block under your right thigh to stabilize your body, if needed. Walk your fingertips back so your shoulders are above your hips. Lift your chest up. Stay here for ten long, deep breaths.

Gently bring yourself out of the split by sitting to the side and making your way back to down dog. Walk your feet up to your hands, roll your torso up to standing and repeat the whole routine up to this point on the other side.

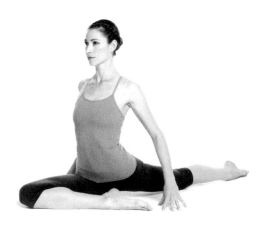

Pigeon Pose

Come into a low lunge with your right leg forward. Gently lower your right leg, still bent at the knee, so that it's resting in front of you in a reverse V. Your right knee will lie on the ground by your right hand and your right foot will lie by your left hand. Rest your hips on the ground or on a blanket or pillow. Sit up as tall as you can in this position. Your hips and shoulders should be working toward facing the front. Stay here for ten long, deep breaths.

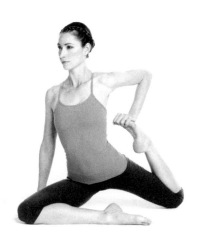

Pigeon Thigh Stretch

If it feels good in your pigeon, bend your back knee and grab hold of the inside of that ankle with your left hand. Gently pull your foot toward your thigh. If there is any pain in the knees, let go, back out of this slowly, and relax.

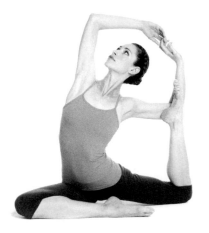

Full Pigeon

If it feels good and there is room to go further, slide your foot into the crook of your elbow and link hands. Stay here for five long, deep breaths. Do the entire routine on the other side.

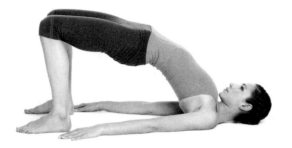

Bridge

Lie down on your back. Bend your knees, grab hold of your ankles, and place your feet on the ground right next to your hips so your knees point straight up. Press your arms into the ground alongside your body and lift your hips straight up. Lift your chest up and slightly behind you. Lengthen your knees in front of you, out from your hips. Try to avoid letting them open out to the sides. Stay here for five long, deep breaths.

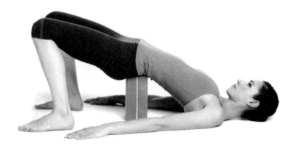

Bridge with Block

For a more restful option place a block under your lower back and stay there for ten long, deep breaths. Favor your exhales slightly more than your inhales to open the back with ease.

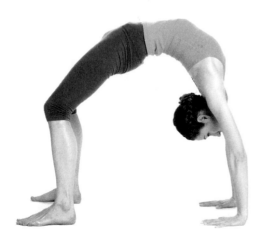

Wheel

Bend your elbows and place the palms of your hands on the ground around your ears. Bring your elbows in so they aren't splaying out to the sides. Lift up in your chest, and begin to straighten your arms. As you straighten your arms keep lifting up through your upper back. Your lower back will arch but keep the focus on your upper back so you don't crunch the lower spine. Press down evenly through both feet and imagine reaching out through your knees. Stay here for five long, deep breaths. To come down, gently tuck your chin into your chest, bend your elbows, and lower down slowly.

Bulging Belly

Whether it's from overeating or drinking too much, or if the tummy is just a problem area for you, some simple yoga moves can help strengthen your core, flatten your belly, and leave you feeling strong and confident. I'm sure you won't be surprised when I say that the best way to accomplish this is to practice regularly. These poses are a great start, but do them every day to strengthen your core from the inside out. We also know that yoga's effect on the mind/body connection helps us to make better food choices, so keeping up a regular practice will put you in the mood to eat healthy and drink less, and as a result also shrink the bulge.

THE BULGING BELLY YOGA CURE

The best way to flatten a bulging tummy is to do a lot of yoga. It's important to engage the entire body to reduce excess weight everywhere. Cultivating a strong core will make it easier to strengthen and tone the rest of your body because you'll be more stable and more energized over all.

This routine is designed to engage the muscles of your entire body and focus the mind. You will be working your core, but you will also be working the big muscles of your thighs and shoulders, and all of the little muscles in between. Stay with your breath and try to move like you are wading through water, using only the muscular effort you need. Do it daily.

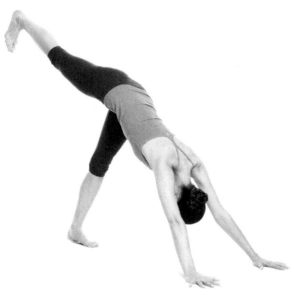

Down Dog Split

Come onto your hands and knees. Spread your fingers wide. Tuck your toes, lift your hips, and press back into a down dog. Reach your heels for the ground, relax your shoulders, and relax your neck and head. Stay here for five long, deep breaths. Inhale and lift your right leg up behind you, keeping your hips square, back toes flexed, and pointed down. Lift from the back of your thigh and lift the leg a little higher. Press down through both hands and out through both feet evenly. Stay here for three long, deep breaths.

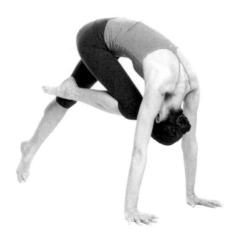

Down Dog Split, Knee to Forehead

From down dog split, lift your hips and belly high and bring your right knee to touch your forehead. Hold here for one long inhale and exhale and press back to down dog split.

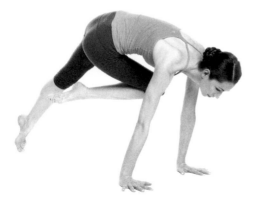

Down Dog Split, Knee Across

From down dog split, keep your hips and belly lifted high, and bring your right knee toward the back of your left upper arm. Hold here for one long inhale and exhale and press back to down dog split. Lower your right leg to down dog and do the three poses with your left leg.

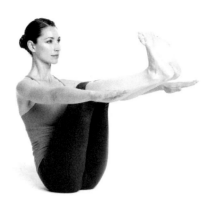

Boat

Sit on your hips, keep your back long, lean back slightly, hold your belly in and up, and lift your legs up so your shins are parallel with the ground. If this is too much pressure, grab hold of your ankles for support. Stay here for ten long, deep breaths.

Leg Raise and Lower Leg

Lie down on your back. Raise your legs straight up in the air. Keeping your lower back relaxed into the ground, slowly lower your legs down to within an inch of the floor and slowly lift them back up. Repeat this movement ten more times. If this movement pinches or hurts your back, sit on the tops of your hands, with your arms under your body and bend your knees slightly. You shouldn't feel any pain in your back when you do this movement, so adjust accordingly. When you're finished, hug your knees into your chest and rock gently from side to side.

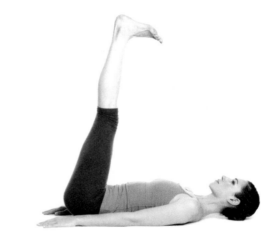

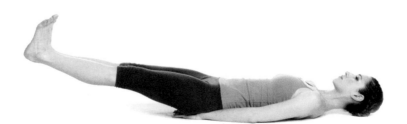

Cellulite

It's pretty universal to want to feel good, strong, and comfortable in your own body. No one wants to live with cellulite. It can make you uncomfortable and make clothing choices tricky, and bikini season terrifying. These swollen fat pockets are caused by unhealthy habits, hormonal changes, bad lymphatic circulation, and toxins deposited under the skin. The good news is, we can do a whole lot to improve our health, minimize or even get rid of cellulite completely, and, most importantly, feel good about ourselves in the process.

THE CELLULITE YOGA CURE

The yoga cure for cellulite is getting your body moving regularly. We'll get the circulation going, move through poses that target the hips, thighs, and butt, and in the process help reduce excess body fat. It's important to practice regularly to gain the most benefit. Reducing processed foods and drinking a lot of water also help to rid the body of toxins that get stored in the fat of your body. Begin the routine with several rounds of sun salutations to get your circulation going and your muscles engaged. Do this routine daily.

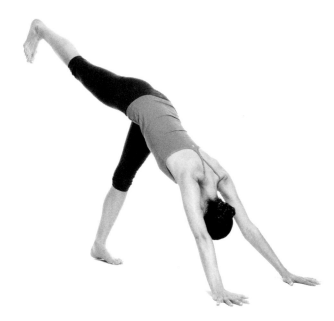

Down Dog Split

Come onto all fours. Spread your fingers wide, tuck your toes, lift your hips and press back into down dog. Inhale and lift your right leg high. Keep your hips square. Press evenly through both hands and feet and lift the back of your right thigh straight up. Stay here for five long, deep breaths.

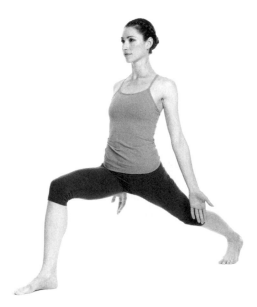

High Lunge Arms Down

From your down dog split, lift your knee in toward your forehead and place your foot on the floor between your hands. Press down through your feet to a standing lunge, reaching your arms behind you and bringing your shoulders in line with your hips. Relax your arms down by your sides, open your palms to face front, and sink your hips low. Stay here for three long, deep breaths.

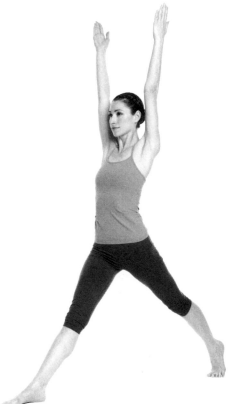

High Lunge Arms and Hips Up

From the previous pose, inhale and lift your hips and arms up. Exhale and lower the arms and hips back down. Repeat this same breath and movement pattern twice more.

High Lunge Twist

From your high lunge with your arms still lifted, exhale and open your torso toward your right, and open your arms. Sink your hips lower. Stay here for three long, deep breaths and come back to your high lunge.

Press your palms down to the ground on either side of your front foot and bring your front leg back and your body into down dog. Gently lower your knees to the ground, unspool into a sitting position, and gently and lie down on your back.

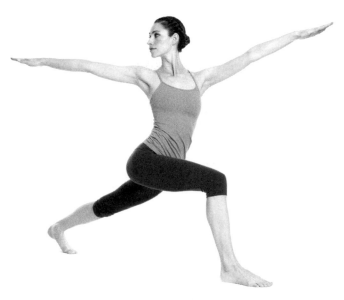

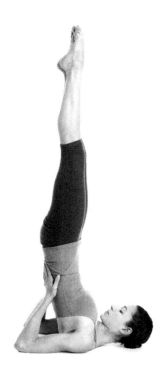

Shoulder Stand

Press your arms down into the floor by your sides, round your back, and bring your feet over your head into a plow pose. (Refer to the pose list for reference in the back of the book if you'd like.) If your neck feels tight, stay there and roll back down to lie on your back slowly. If your neck feels good, press your palms into your back so the tops of your fingers point up. Wiggle your elbows closer together and scoot your hands down your back closer to your shoulders. Lift the backs of your legs straight up so your body is in one straight line. Stay here for twenty long, deep breaths. Either close your eyes or keep your gaze softly rested on your belly button.

Chill the *&@# Out

Sometimes we're overworked, sometimes we're overtired, sometimes we're too stressed, and sometimes we just need to chill out! When your body holds on to stress, it's harder to relax, even when we have chill-out time. These simple yoga poses can undo stresses we hold in the body and mind so we can fully relax with ease.

THE CHILL THE *&@# OUT YOGA CURE

When tension builds in us, it stays with us until we do something about it. We often store tension in our sides, spine, hips, as well as our minds, so we'll send it on its way with this routine. Do it anytime you need to take a chill pill, side-effect free!

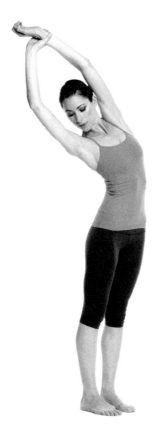

Standing Side Opener

Stand with your feet parallel to each other, shoulders aligned with your hips. Inhale and reach your arms out and up. Grab your left wrist with your right hand. Gently pull your left arm up with your right hand. Let your torso naturally arch over to your right side. Stay here for three long, deep breaths and then work the other side.

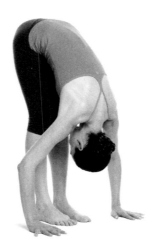

Standing Forward Bend

From the previous pose, stand straight and comfortably. Exhale and bend your trunk forward over your legs. Let your head and neck relax and hang heavy. Press your fingertips on the ground. If your hamstrings feel tight keep a slight bend in your knees to give them some more space to relax and open.

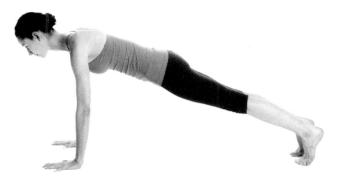

Plank

Move from forward bend to letting your hands rest on the floor under your shoulders. Press your palms firmly into the ground, while you step your feet back to the top of a push-up position. Lengthen your body, stretching forward to the top of your head, keeping your neck long, and push your heels back. Keep your stomach nice and strong and lift the front of your thighs up. Stay here for five long, deep breaths. If this is too intense feel free to gently lower your knees to the floor and let it support some of your weight. Always make sure you can breathe easily during this pose.

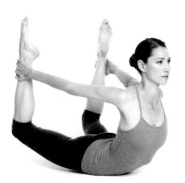

Bow

From plank, bend your elbows and slowly lower your body to the ground. Bend your knees, and reaching around from the outside of both legs, grab hold of the outside of your ankles with your hands. This action will lift your body and open your spine. Only press as far as you can while still breathing easily. Stay here for five long, deep breaths then slowly lower down. Take a few breaths as you just lie comfortable on the floor.

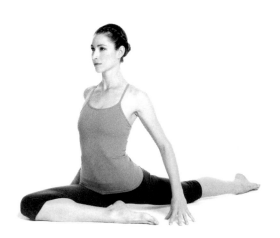

Pigeon

Get onto all fours then bend your right knee and gently move it forward and lie it on its side in front of you (it should make an inverted V). Straighten your left leg behind you and sink your hips into the ground. If they don't reach the ground sit on a pillow or a block. Turn your hips and shoulders so they both face your front. Do your best to sit up straight here. Stay here for ten long, deep breaths. Do the other side.

Cold Repair

Colds can be repaired with yoga. That's the good news. The even better news is that the more yoga you practice the less you'll get colds in the first place. A regular yoga practice will strengthen your immunity. Your yoga practice and these additional breathing techniques can cleanse the body and the sinuses, leaving you feeling refreshed and relieved even during the worst of colds.

THE COLD REPAIR YOGA CURE

This routine is designed to strengthen your immunity, clear your nasal passages, balance your nervous system, and calm you. So even if your cold persists a little longer, doing this routine will make you more comfortable while you're sniffling your way back to good health.

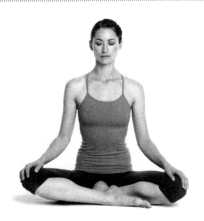

Breath of Fire

Sitting tall and comfortably, hands resting on your lap, close your eyes and take a long and deep inhale. Exhale all of the air out. Begin to breathe rapidly in and out through the nose. Pick up the pace if you can and keep your inhales and exhales even. Continue for one minute. After a minute slow down your inhales and exhales gradually until you come back to long and deep breathing. Gently open your eyes.

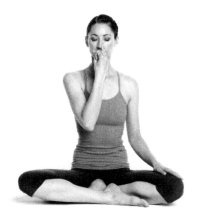

Alternate Nostril Breathing

Sit up tall. Take your right hand and curl down your index and middle finger into your palm. You'll be left with your ring finger and your thumb, which is a perfect space for your nose in between.

Press your ring finger over your left nostril and inhale for four counts through your right nostril. Close off your right nostril with your thumb so both sides of your nostrils are closed. Hold all the air in for four counts. Release your ring finger and let all the air out your left nostril for four counts. Reverse this pattern and repeat for three to five minutes.

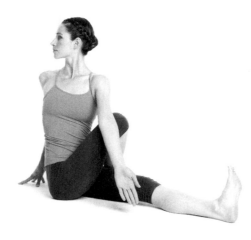

Seated Spine Twist

Extend your left leg out in front of you. Hug your right knee in toward your chest and place your right foot on the ground next to your left hip, crossing it over your left leg. Inhale and lift your left arm straight up. As you exhale, cross your arm over your right leg. Press your right fingertips on the ground behind your hips. Inhale and lift your torso up tall, exhale and twist your torso further to your right. Repeat this same movement and breathing pattern twice more. Gently reverse the twist of your torso to release. Switch legs and do the same thing on the other side.

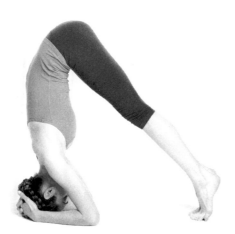

Headstand Prep

Sit on your heels. Interlace your fingers loosely and place them on the ground. Place the top of your head on the ground so your fingers hold the back of your head. Stay here for a few breaths to get comfortable in the position. If this feels uncomfortable, come back to sit on your heels. Stay here for a few breaths. If you are comfortable, tuck your toes and straighten your legs. Stay here for ten long, deep breaths and when you are ready come out of it gently, lower your knees to the ground, and relax in child's pose.

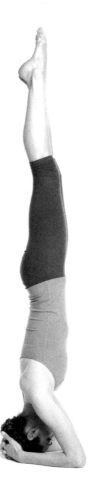

Headstand

If you want to move on to a full headstand, start to walk your feet in toward your body so your hips line up over your shoulders and your back is straight up and down. Stay here for a few breaths. If you are comfortable here bend one knee in and bring your heel to your hip. Bring it back down and try the other leg. If you are steady with one leg try both legs at the same time. When your heels are pulled in toward your hips, slowly extend your legs straight up. Stay for twenty long, deep breaths if you can. When you are ready to come down, slowly lower one leg at a time and rest in child's pose for a few breaths.

Couch-stination

Ever get stuck on the couch, literally? What begins as a harmless moment of total body and mind relaxation can quickly develop into cozy nesting that takes a sudden turn for the worse into zombie-like vegetation without much hope for a snappy return back to our normal, energetic selves. Once we hit the zombie state of couch-stination we literally get stuck in the couch. The cushions and pillows swallow us up like quicksand and we are done for. TV movies, snacks, magazines, books, everything you could ever want is within arm's reach, so no wonder it's so easy to get buried in the couch.

THE COUCH-STINATION YOGA CURE

The only cure for couch-stination is to find just a bit of inspiration to begin some simple and mindful movements. Know that starting off slow will help bring vitality back into your body and energize your whole system. Once you begin these simple movements designed to increase circulation and range of motion, you'll be back to your usual self in no time. If you are suffering from couch-stination and have even the slightest desire to get some movement and energy back into your system, this routine can help. And the best part is you don't even have to get off the couch to do it. Fair warning: after you do this routine you may be inspired to go for a walk and enjoy some non-couch-related activities.

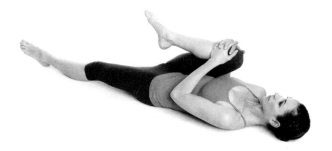

Reclining Single Knee Hug

Lie down on your back. Hug your right knee gently into your chest. With each exhale, draw your knee closer to your right shoulder. Stay here for five long, deep breaths.

Reclined Single Knee Hug Twist

From your reclining knee hug, cross your right knee over your body toward your left hip. Open your arms out on either side of you, laying your palms flat on the couch if you can. If it's too small a space, just keep your hands loosely folded at your hips. Look toward your right. Stay here for ten long, deep breaths. Do the other side starting with the reclining knee hug.

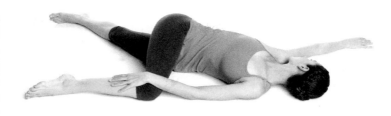

Half Happy Baby

Still lying down on your back, hug your right knee into your chest. Point the bottom of your foot straight up. Grab the outside edge of your right foot with your right hand and press your knee down toward the couch with the strength of your right arm. Stay here for five long, deep breaths then do the other side.

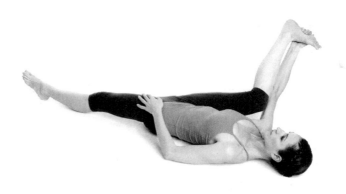

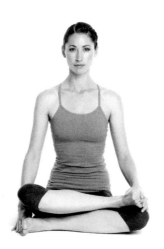

Seated Ankle to Knee

Sit up tall. Bend your knees and fold your legs toward you as if you were coming into a seated meditation. Lift your right leg and stack it on top of your left leg so your right ankle is on top of your left knee and your right knee is on top of your left ankle. Stay here for ten long, deep breaths then do the other side.

Depression

If you are suffering from severe depression, seeing a physician is a great place to begin. But whether you simply have a case of the blues, or a more daunting depression cloud is looming over your head, fortunately there are some simple practices that can hopefully lighten the load quite a bit. Regular practice resting the mind on the breath eases anxiety and raises GABA levels in the brain, sending depression on its dark, sad way. The noncompetitive, rhythmic aspects of yoga are also comforting and go a long way toward healing the whole person.

THE DEPRESSION YOGA CURE

The yoga cure for depression is simply to practice regularly, even when you don't feel like it. A little bit of yoga is better than nothing. The more you practice, the better you'll feel.

This routine, like many of the others, is designed to calm and focus the mind and simultaneously settle tension in the body, while strengthening the body from the inside out. It also challenges your balance a bit so we can have a little fun! Do it daily.

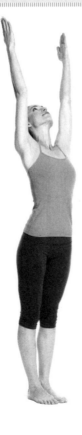

Standing Arm Reach

Inhale and lift your arms out to your sides and up, filling all the space with your breath and your movement. Relax your tailbone and lift your chest. Keep your shoulders relaxed and down and look up while keeping your face and your forehead relaxed.

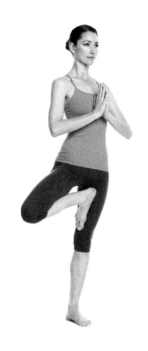

Tree Pose

Stand tall and comfortably with your feet parallel and a few inches apart. Shift your weight into your left leg. Bend your right knee into your chest and hug your shin with your hands. Grab hold of your right ankle with your right hand and press the bottom of your right foot into your left inner thigh. Keep pressure going both ways, from your thigh into your foot and your foot into your thigh, just like a magnet stuck to a fridge. Either stay here with your hand holding your ankle for balance, or reach your arms straight up. Stay here for five long, deep breaths. Try the same thing on your other side.

Warrior 3

Hug your left shin into your chest, then extend it straight back behind you so it's parallel to the ground. Flex your left foot and point the toes down. Bring your fingertips to the ground to stabilize yourself. Reach your arms out in front of you so your body is in a straight line from your fingertips all the way down your back and out through your left heel. Stay here for three long, deep breaths. Bend both knees slightly and again hug your left shin into your chest and place your left foot next to your right to come back to standing. Do the same thing on the other side, starting with tree pose first.

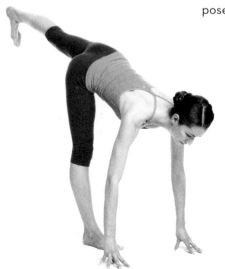

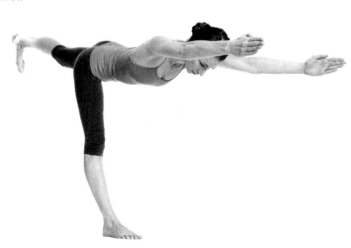

Diabetes

Yoga practice has been found beneficial for helping people with diabetes. Findings from several studies indicate that yoga may benefit diabetes patients by reducing body fat, helping with blood sugar control, fighting insulin resistance, and improving nerve function. Yoga reduces stress, which reduces levels of glucose, and possibly improves insulin response. Yoga also helps regulate blood pressure and cholesterol levels, which plays a big role in the development of diabetes and its related complications. Yoga is also beneficial for stimulating pancreatic function, which secretes hormones that affect the level of sugar in the blood.

THE DIABETES YOGA CURE

The yoga cure for diabetes is to first prevent getting this sickness by keeping a regular practice and healthy lifestyle. If you already have diabetes, our aim together is to prevent further complications from developing and to improve the functions of the body's systems. A regular practice can help bring your body back to working for, not against you. Do this routine daily, along with sun salutations, to get your entire body moving fluidly.

Plow

Start lying down, press your arms down into the floor by your sides, round your back, and bring your feet over your head into a plow pose. If your neck feels pretty tight in plow, stay there for a little longer and roll back down to lie on your back slowly.

Shoulder Stand

If your neck feels good in plow, press your palms into your back so the tops of your fingers point up. Wiggle your elbows closer together and scoot your hands down your back closer to your shoulders. Lift the backs of your legs straight up so your body is in one straight line. Stay here for twenty long, deep breaths. Either close your eyes or keep your gaze softly rested on your belly button.

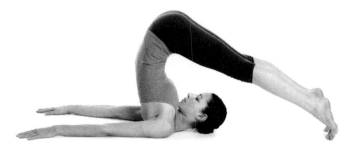

Droopy Shoulders

All day long our shoulders tend to droop further and further forward. If we continue this drooping day after day for years of our lives we will end up all hunched over, shrinking our size and causing our bodies a lot of totally preventable tension. Whether your shoulders sag from computer use, poor posture, or because you're just hanging out trying to look cool, it's way more cool to have good posture and be able to stand up tall throughout your entire life. If you're hunched forward, you're going to miss a lot of the action in life.

THE DROOPY SHOULDERS YOGA CURE

The yoga cure for droopy shoulders is to open the chest and get those shoulders down and rested back, where they belong. Repetition is key. Just because you do this routine once, and you're standing up taller immediately after, doesn't mean you're finished there. Keep up the yoga and shoulder opener poses to have perfect posture and tension-free shoulders that you can walk around proudly with for years.

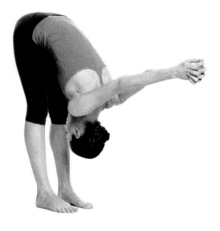

Standing Forward Bend Shoulder Opener

Stand comfortably with your feet a few inches apart. Inhale deeply. As you exhale, gently fold your torso forward over your legs. Interlace your hands behind you and let your arms fall over your back. If your hamstrings feel tense, bend your knees slightly and rest your belly on your thighs. Relax deeper into the pose with each exhale. Begin to lengthen your exhales a bit more than your inhales; this will encourage the body to open and the mind to settle. Stay here for five long, deep breaths.

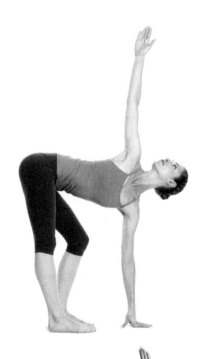

Back Lengthener, Easy Twist

From your standing forward bend, unlace your hands and release your fingertips to the ground. Press your left fingertips into the ground a couple inches in front of your feet, soften your left knee, open your torso toward your right, lengthening your right arm back and straight up over your shoulders. Simultaneously, lengthen out through your tailbone and through the top of your head. Stay here for three long, deep breaths. Do the other side.

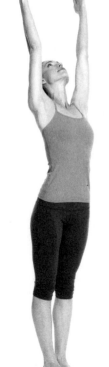

Standing Arm Reach

Now bring both fingertips to the ground, bend your knees slightly, let your head hang heavy and roll up to standing, one vertebra at a time. When your head is lifted, inhale and lift your arms out and up. Relax your tailbone and lift your chest. As you exhale relax and let your arms gently float down to your sides. Repeat this twice more.

Exhaustion

Keeping up with our busy schedules and all the activities of our lives can lead to exhaustion, especially if we are spreading ourselves too thin. A regular yoga practice will help you take an honest look at how you spend your time, and naturally guide you toward filling your days with activities that inspire and fill you with energy, instead of activities that drain you and cause stress and tension to build up.

Your attitude toward your day is a huge factor in your energy level. Sometimes, we just need to "get through" big stretches of some activity that we really aren't excited about. Working hard on something you don't like usually leads us right to exhaustion. When you wake up each day excited about what it might bring, your energy levels will skyrocket, no matter how much busyness the day brings. To flip your mood from dread-filled to excited, practice these simple yoga poses regularly and you'll be re-inspired and energized in no time. If a lack of sleep is causing your exhaustion, yoga can also help ease your body and mind so you can sleep great at night. All you have to do is make the time to practice and take care of yourself.

THE EXHAUSTION YOGA CURE

The yoga cure for exhaustion is simply getting up and doing these simple yoga poses. A little gentle movement will awaken your entire system, and leave you with a fresh and lasting energy that you can take with you.

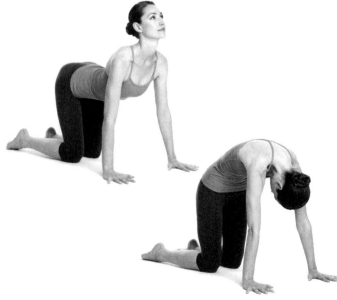

Cat/Cow

Come onto all fours, on your hands and knees. Spread your fingers wide like you are digging into some nice, wet sand. Make sure your wrists are right under your shoulders and knees under your hips. Have a nice, neutral spine that is straight and long, not arched or curved. Bring your attention to your breath. Lengthen and deepen your inhales and exhales. Take five long, deep breaths here in this neutral place.

Now beginning to move with your breath on your next inhale, drop your belly toward the ground, allow your spine to curve, and look up (cow pose). As you inhale, round your back and look inward (cat pose).

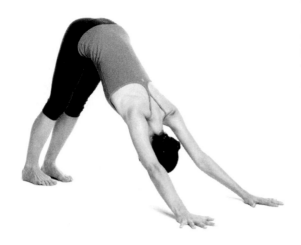

Down Dog

From all fours, tuck your toes, lift your hips, and press back into down dog. Reach your heels toward the ground. Relax your shoulders toward the ground and relax your head and neck. Stay here for five long, deep breaths.

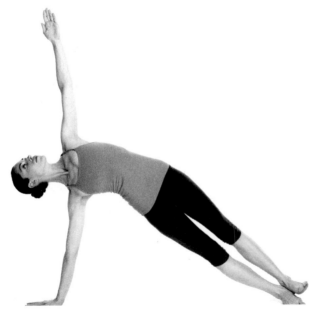

Side Plank

From your down dog, roll your torso out into a plank pose. Lift your hips, press down with your right hand, roll to the outside edge of your right foot, and open your torso toward the left. Extend your left arm straight up and look up to your fingers. Stay here for three long, deep breaths and do the other side.

Fear Factor

There are a whole set of poses in yoga to help us deal with our fears. They are the ones where we go upside down, into the unknown, and have to abandon control just for a moment, before we get a really nice release and the enjoyable sensation of experiencing a new situation. Backbends and inversions are often associated with fear in yoga because our perspective becomes something completely different than when we are grounded and standing on our own two feet. It's a nice physical way to work out fears in our bodies that can also translate into dealing with fears in our lives. So whether you have a fear of going upside down in yoga, or a fear of entering into a new stage in your life, backbends and inversions can be of great use! You have to learn to feel your way through the poses and trust that you are strong enough to get through them, and above all, allow yourself to have some fun. It's yoga, after all. It's meant to be enjoyable . . . just like life!

THE FEAR FACTOR YOGA CURE

The yoga cure for getting over your fears is trying new yoga poses, especially those in which you are upside down or backwards. When we go into the unknown with our bodies, we can do it in the rest of our lives. This routine also reminds us to have fun, and not to worry about being perfect and in control the whole time. Falling is totally fine in yoga. Go ahead, have a fall. Just go easy on yourself and have a good time!

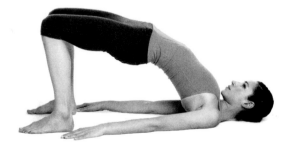

Bridge

Lie down on your back. Bend your knees and press the bottoms of your feet into the ground next to the bottom of your hips so your knees point straight up. Press your arms down by your sides and use them to help you lift your hips and chest up and off the ground. Stay here for five long, deep breaths.

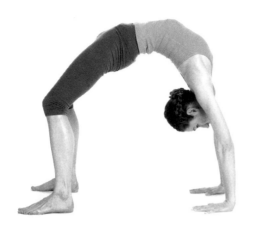

Wheel

Bend your elbows and press your palms into the ground by your ears. Press into your palms firmly and begin to lift the chest up. Straighten your arms only as much as you can while keeping the chest lifted and being able to breathe easily. Lengthen your knees forward and keep your spine long. Stay here for five long, deep breaths. To come down, tuck your chin in toward your chest, bend your elbows, and slowly lower down.

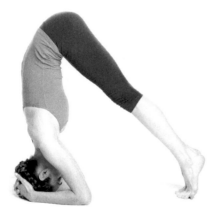

Headstand Prep

Sit on your heels. Interlace your fingers loosely and place them on the ground. Place the top of your head on the ground so your fingers hold the back of your head. Stay here for a few breaths to get comfortable in the position. If this is too hard or feels uncomfortable, back out of it and come back to sit on your heels.

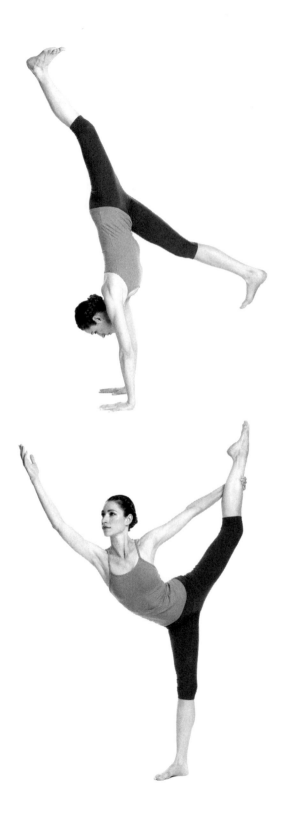

Handstand Rocks

Stand on your right leg, tip your weight forward so your left leg extends back behind you and your fingertips come to the ground. Press your palms firmly on the ground under your shoulders. Straighten your arms. Keep the left leg lifted and rock forward and back, just starting to get your hips over your shoulders. Start to take small hops on your right leg. When you hop up, lift your left leg high so your hips are over your shoulders and keep your right leg dangling down so your legs will be in an L shape. Keep breathing through the entire movement. Inhale as you rock or lightly hop up, and exhale as you release. Try the other side.

Dancer

Shift your weight onto your right leg. Bend your left knee and grab the inside of your left calf with your left hand. Gently press your foot into your hand to open your back. Reach your right arm straight up. Stay here for five long, deep breaths. Try the other side.

Fibromyalgia

According to the American College of Rheumatology, fibromyalgia affects 3 to 6 million Americans, mostly women of childbearing age, but children, the elderly, and men can also be affected. Fibromyalgia sufferers experience long-term, bodywide pain and tender points in joints, muscles, tendons, and other soft tissues. Fibromyalgia has also been linked to fatigue, sleep problems, headache, depression, and anxiety.

Yet again, yoga can help. According to a study conducted by James Carson, PhD, at the Oregon Health and Science University, yoga exercise may have the power to combat fibromyalgia. The researchers enrolled fifty-three female study subjects who had been previously diagnosed with fibromyalgia. The women were randomly assigned to two research groups. The first group participated in an eight-week yoga program, which included gentle poses, meditation, breathing exercises, and group discussions. The control group received standard medication treatments for fibromyalgia. Following the completion of the yoga program, comparison of the groups revealed that yoga appears to assist in combating a number of serious fibromyalgia symptoms, including pain, fatigue, stiffness, poor sleep, depression, poor memory, anxiety, and poor balance. Pain was reduced in the yoga group by an average of 24 percent, fatigue by 30 percent, and depression by 42 percent.

THE FIBROMYALGIA YOGA CURE

With any cure, especially when dealing with physical pain and range of motion limitations, attention, care, and patience are not just useful, but crucial. Stay easy in your body when you practice and the yoga can have the most impact.

This routine is designed to work through aches and pains very gently with deep breathing and relaxation of the muscles. Go slowly and make sure to pay attention to the breath so you can release tension on your exhales without forcing or straining the body.

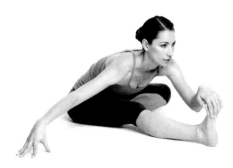

Seated One Leg Forward Bend

Sit up tall. Extend your right leg forward and flex your right foot. Bend your left foot in toward your body so your knee relaxes out toward the left side a bit. Inhale and extend your arms straight up. Exhale and fold your torso over your right leg. Grab your right toes with your left hand and press your right fingertips on the ground beside your right leg. Extend the left side of your back out so that it's straight and long. Stay here for ten long, deep breaths.

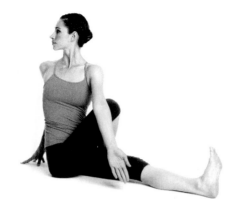

Seated Spine Twist

Gently bring your torso to sit upright. Hug your right knee into your chest and place your right foot on the ground across and outside your left leg so your knee is pointing straight up. Inhale your left arm straight up and lengthen through your torso. As you exhale, cross your arm over your right thigh. Press your right finger-tips into the ground behind your hips. As you inhale, lengthen the spine tall, as you exhale, twist further. Repeat this breathing and movement pattern three more times and slowly reverse your torso to the left side for a countertwist. Repeat the single-leg forward bend and the seated spine twist on the other side.

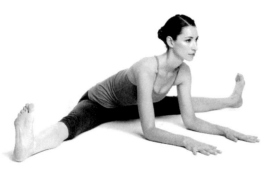

Seated Wide Leg Straddle

Sit up tall and open your legs to the sides until you feel a little tension, but not so much that it is uncomfortable. Walk your hands forward between your legs and keep your torso long. Stay here for ten long, deep breaths favoring the exhales a bit more than the inhales to encourage tension to release.

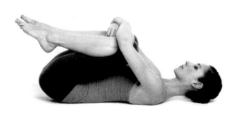

Reclining Knee Hug

Gently lie down on your back. Hug both knees into your chest. Wrap your arms around your shins and slowly rock side to side, releasing your lower back on the ground. Stay here for ten long, deep breaths.

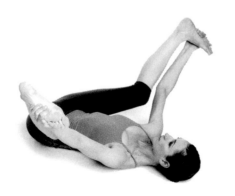

Happy Baby

Lie down on your back. Draw your knees into your chest. Grab the outsides of your feet with your hands so the bottoms of your feet point straight up. Gently pull your knees down toward the ground outside your torso using the strength of your arms. If it feels good rock carefully from side to side to open your back and hips even more. Stay here for ten long, deep breaths.

Flu

Your yoga practice will build up your immunity so you won't get as sick as often, and hopefully not at all, but when the flu does strike, the body aches, chills, and fever are no fun. When you have the flu, the last thing you may want to do is get out of bed, but some simple yoga poses can help bring your body back to health. These very simple poses can help you feel better faster than burying yourself under the covers. Simple inversions in yoga stimulate your lymphatic system, which acts as a waste disposal system for your entire body. Targeting your lymphatic system with yoga will cleanse your body, ridding it of any lingering viruses from the flu. Yoga poses that use gentle twists increase blood flow to your spleen, fight against infections, and cleanse the blood.

THE FLU YOGA CURE

This simple routine is designed to relax and restore your entire system from the inside out and calm your mind at the same time. When your mind is relaxed, your body can bring you back to optimal health quickly and easily. When your body is at ease it can do its job a whole lot better than when it is filled with tension and anxiety.

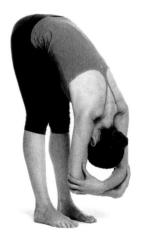

Standing Forward Bend Elbow Hold

Stand up tall with your feet under your hips and parallel to each other. Bend your knees slightly and fold your torso over your legs. Grab opposite elbows, forming a square, and let your head and neck hang heavy. Stay here for five long, deep breaths. If it feels good, gently sway your torso from side to side.

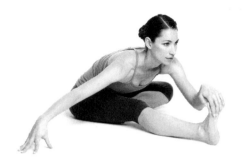

Seated One-Leg Forward Bend

Sit up tall with your legs extended in front of you. Bend your left knee in toward your body, and open your knee out to the side so the bottom of your foot rests on your right upper thigh. As you inhale, reach your arms straight up. As you exhale, lengthen your torso forward over your right leg. Grab your right foot with your left hand and press your right fingertips into the floor outside your right leg. Lengthen the left side of your back so that it feels long and reaches across your right leg. Stay here for ten long, deep breaths. Repeat on the other side.

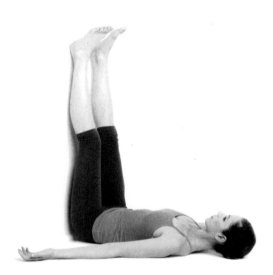

Legs Up the Wall

Sit facing a wall. Bring the bottom of your hips right up to the wall. Lie down so your torso is perpendicular to the wall. Raise your legs and rest them on the wall. Stay here for five minutes.

Foot Cramps

Foot cramps can be a painful side effect of simply wearing shoes all day long, especially uncomfortable ones. In yoga, foot cramps can also happen because your body might not be used to being worked in certain ways. Yoga definitely works out the feet, strengthening and stretching all the little muscles that hold your feet up, and which in turn hold you up all day long.

THE FOOT CRAMPS YOGA CURE

Working the feet with some simple yoga poses is great for preventing these cramps, and also for relieving pain when you are in the middle of a cramp. If your feet cramp up during a class, try sitting on your heels with knees in front of you and your toes tucked until the cramping fades. To prevent cramps and strengthen the feet do the following routine regularly.

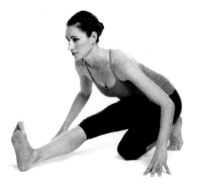

Runner's Stretch

Come into a low lunge with your right foot forward. Tuck the toes of your back foot under and lower your back knee to the ground. Shift your hips back to sit on your back heel. Your right leg should be straight in front of you. Relax your torso over your front leg. Stay here for five long, deep breaths. Bring yourself back to your lunge and do the same thing with the other leg.

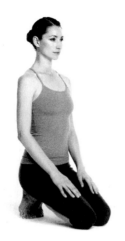

Sit on Heels, Toes Tucked

Sit on your heels so your shoulders are aligned with your hips. Next, tuck your toes and sit on your heels so you can get a nice stretch for the arches of your feet. Relax your hands on your thighs and stay here for ten long, deep breaths.

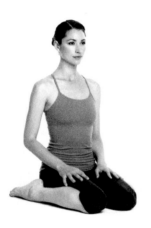

Hero

Come into a kneeling position with your knees directly under your hips. Press the tops of your feet down and into the ground. Carefully sit your hips down until they meet the ground between your legs. If your hips don't make it to the ground without straining your knees, sit on a pillow, blanket, or yoga block. Point your knees forward and feel them "reaching" in that direction. Stay here for ten long, deep breaths.

Hero Reclined

If you can sit on the ground easily in your hero without a pillow and you feel like there is more room to work within this pose, slowly lower your back to the ground and reach your arms overhead. Throughout the pose, you should continue to press down into the ground through the tops of your feet and reach forward through your knees. Stay here for ten long, deep breaths and slowly bring yourself up and out of the pose.

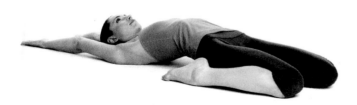

Hangover

When you are hung low by a hangover the only thing you want is for it to go away. The last thing you may be thinking of for a cure is yoga, but it is one of the best hangover helpers around. My Saturday midmorning class is usually packed with a fair number of people suffering from self-induced dehydration, dizziness, and shakiness from having too much to drink the night before. They flock to yoga because they know that after a little over an hour of down dogs, twists, and inversions, their hangover will be cured.

THE HANGOVER YOGA CURE

The best way to cure a hangover is to not get one in the first place. Drinking until you get drunk is not really all that fun. With a regular yoga practice, you might start to notice yourself enjoying one glass of wine, but not the whole bottle. Your tolerance for alcohol might even lower quite a bit when your body gets super clean from all the yoga. (I speak from experience here. Yoga changes you in all sorts of ways. Some you see coming. Some come as complete curveballs.)

When hangovers do happen, it's good to have yoga on your side. Twisting yoga poses literally wring out toxins from your body (alcohol included), get digestion moving, and keep the blood flow fresh. Yoga also improves circulation and helps the body produce a fresh supply of blood. Headstands are well known to cure headaches and hangovers. Depending on the degree of your yoga experience and the severity of your hangover, please practice headstand wisely and carefully. Do this routine when you're hung over. If you are doing this routine more than once a month, do more yoga, less drinking.

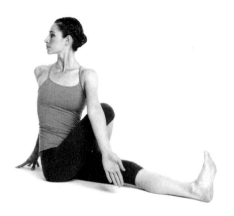

Seated Spine Twist

Come into a comfortable seated position. Hug your right knee into your chest and place your right foot on the ground across and outside your right leg. Take a long, deep inhale through your nose. Exhale through your mouth. Repeat this breathing pattern twice more. Inhale with your left arm straight up. As you exhale, rest your left hand on your right knee. Press your right fingertips into the ground behind your hips. Inhale and lift your torso and chest up. Exhale and twist your torso toward the right. Repeat this breathing and movement pattern twice more. Gently bring your torso back to center. Do the same thing on the other side.

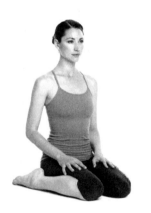

Hero

Stand on your knees with your shoulders aligned above your hips. Press your thumbs into the backs of your knees and move your calves out to the sides. Press into the ground with the tops of your feet, especially at the edges, near your pinkies. Sit your hips back between your legs, either on the ground or on a pillow. If you feel anything in your knees, sit up on a pillow, don't force your hips to meet the floor. Rest your shoulders above your hips and rest your palms on your thighs. Stay here for ten long, deep breaths. This pose stimulates digestion and calms the mind.

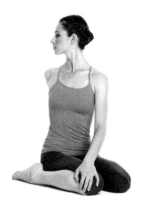

Hero Twist

Grab your right knee with your left hand. Press your right fingertips into the ground behind your hips. Inhale and lift your torso and chest up. Exhale and twist toward your right. Repeat this breathing and movement pattern twice more. Do the same thing on the other side.

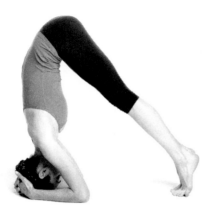

Headstand Prep/Headstand

When hung over, headstand at your own risk. Even if you are an expert headstander, your ability is a little skewed when you are hung over. If you are attempting your first headstand, it's probably best to start on a day when you're 100 percent sober.

Sit on your heels. Interlace your fingers loosely and place them on the ground. Place the top of your head on the ground so your fingers hold the back of your head. Stay here for a few breaths to get comfortable in the position. If this feels uncomfortable, back out of it and come back to sit on your heels. If you are comfortable, tuck your toes and straighten your legs. Stay here for ten long, deep breaths and when you are ready do come out of it gently lower your knees to the ground and relax in child's pose.

If you want to move onto a full headstand, start to walk your feet in toward your body so your hips line up over your shoulders and your back is vertical. Stay here for a few breaths. If you are comfortable, bend one knee in and bring your heel to your hip. Bring it back down and try the other leg. If you are steady with one leg, try both legs at the same time. When your heels are pulled in toward your hips, slowly extend your legs straight up. Stay for twenty long, deep breaths if you can. When you are ready to come down, slowly lower one leg at a time and rest in child's pose for a few breaths.

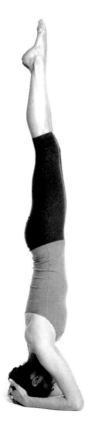

High Blood Pressure

Hypertension, commonly known as high blood pressure, happens when the pressure in your arteries gets high enough that it endangers the function of your heart and other organs. Some factors that play a role in developing high blood pressure: being overweight, smoking, stress, lack of physical activity, and too much alcohol consumption (more than one to two drinks per day). Hypertension can lead to kidney infection, malfunctioning of the endocrine glands, and problems with the arteries. Chronic hypertension may lead to heart attack, heart failure, or a stroke. Often, but not solely, caused by stress, high blood pressure frequently goes undetected and is known as a silent killer.

Not to get all scary on you, but high blood pressure is serious business, and so are your stress levels. Make sure you're doing your yoga daily and living a healthy lifestyle—and, of course, under a physician's care, which together with your practice can keep your blood pressure in check.

THE HIGH BLOOD PRESSURE YOGA CURE

Moving through these calming yoga poses and breathing techniques can lower blood pressure. Some simple inversions are also useful because they trigger several internal reflexes that reduce blood pressure. Regular practice is necessary to achieve lasting benefits. Again, check with your physician before beginning any physical exercise program.

REAL-LIFE CURES: Todd's Blood Pressure and Cholesterol Drop

When Todd began practicing yoga, he had high blood pressure, high cholesterol, high stress, and he was about fifty pounds overweight. He had recently relocated to New York City for his job and had found his way to Strala for yoga. After becoming convinced that regular practice would be the way to go to kick-start a healthy lifestyle, Todd really became hooked when he started to notice a big difference in his stress levels and mood after a few weeks of practicing several times a week. At a routine checkup with his doctor he learned that his blood pressure and cholesterol had dropped to healthy levels. In just a few months he also lost thirty pounds. Todd continues practicing yoga several times a week to manage his health, weight, and stress.

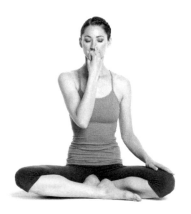

Alternate Nostril Breathing

Sit up tall, however you can sit comfortably. Take your right hand and curl down your index and middle finger into your palm. You'll be left with your ring finger and your thumb, which is a perfect space for your nose to rest between. This hand position will help you alternate between nostrils as you inhale and exhale.

Press your ring finger over your left nostril and inhale for four counts through your right nostril. Close off your right nostril with your thumb so both sides of your nostrils are closed. Hold all the air in for four counts. Release your ring finger and let all the air out your left nostril for four counts. Reverse this pattern starting with inhaling through the left nostril, holding both closed, and exhaling out the right side. Repeat this breathing pattern for three to five minutes.

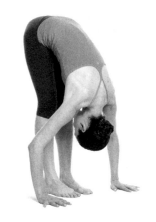

Standing Forward Bend

Exhale and bend your trunk forward over your legs. Let your head and neck relax and hang heavy. If your hamstrings feel tight keep a slight bend in your knees to give them some more space to relax and open. Press your fingertips on the ground.

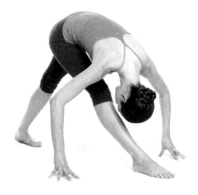

Single Leg Forward Bend

From the last pose, press your fingertips into the floor on either side of your legs. Step your left leg back a couple feet behind your right leg. Straighten both legs and fold your torso over your front leg. If your front leg doesn't straighten easily, bend it enough so your fingers can press into the ground. Stay here for ten long, deep breaths and then repeat on the other side.

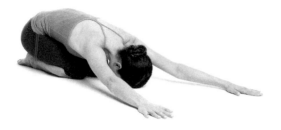

Child's Pose

Gently come onto all fours. Relax your hips and sit back on your heels. Rest your forehead on the ground and breathe deeply into your back. Stay here for five long, deep breaths.

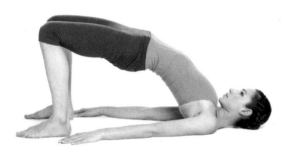

Bridge

Lie down on your back. Bend your knees and press the bottoms of your feet into the ground next to your body so your knees point straight up. Press your arms down by your sides and lift your hips and chest up. Stay here for five long, deep breaths.

Hot Flashes

Either caused by hormonal conditions, or most usually menopause, hot flashes are a sudden, intense hot feeling, possibly followed with sweating, anxiety, weakness, and an increased heartbeat. Not something that we would wish upon ourselves for sure!

Researchers at the University of Massachusetts Medical School in Worcester enrolled 110 women with at least five or more bothersome hot flashes each day. The women were assigned to two groups. One participated in weekly two-and-a-half-hour mindfulness classes focused on body awareness, meditation, and stretching. Women in the second group were put on a wait list with no intervention. By the time the women in the first group had finished the mindfulness program they were less stressed and anxious and were no longer considered out of the normal range for those symptoms. They also slept better, rated their quality of life higher, and were less bothered by their hot flashes. In 2002, the Women's Health Initiative study found that hormone therapy used to relieve menopause symptoms increased women's risk of stroke as well as breast and ovarian cancers, so looking to alternative means for a cure is a good idea.

THE HOT FLASHES YOGA CURE

To cool it down and ward off hot flashes, try this routine at least three times a week. The routine will bring your body back to a neutral, chilled-out state.

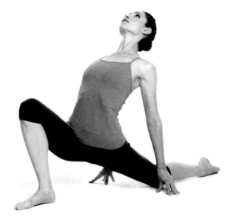

Low Lunge, Back Knee Down Arch

Come into a low lunge with your right leg forward and your left leg back. Sink your hips low toward the ground. Take three long, deep breaths here. Gently lower your back knee to the floor. Walk your fingertips back so they are under your shoulders. Sink your hips forward, drop your tailbone down, and arch your chest up. Stay here for five long, deep breaths.

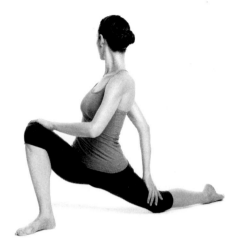

Low Lunge, Back Knee Down, Twist

From your previous pose, twist your torso to your right. Press your left hand on your right thigh and rest your right hand on your back leg. Open your chest toward your left side and look over your right shoulder. Stay here for three long, deep breaths.

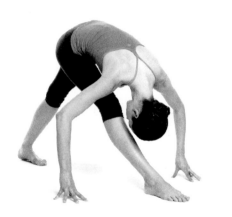

Single Leg Forward Bend

From the last pose, press your fingertips into the floor by either side of your legs. Step your left leg back a couple feet behind your right leg. Straighten both legs and fold your torso over your front leg. If your front leg doesn't straighten easily, bend it enough so your fingers can press into the ground. Stay here for ten long, deep breaths and then repeat on the other side.

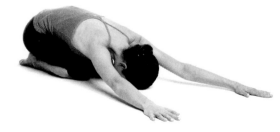

Child's Pose

Gently come onto all fours. Relax your hips and sit back on your heels. Rest your forehead on the ground and breathe deeply into your back. Stay here for five long, deep breaths. Perform the routine on the other side.

Jiggly Thighs

Jiggly thighs may not be the most severe medical condition to be cured by yoga, but toning up makes you stronger, leaner, lighter, and more efficient. It just feels better. When you practice regularly, yoga has a way of sculpting a fantastic, healthy body from the inside out, leaving you with a "firm foundation," and a vibrant body to live in.

THE JIGGLY THIGHS YOGA CURE

The cure for jiggly thighs has a few parts. Probably even more important than the physical benefits of these poses that strengthen your lower body is the harmonious mental state that your regular practice will give you. Food choices are everything when it comes to how your body is shaped, and when you are feeling calm and settled after regular yoga practice you are much more likely to reach for the kale-and-cucumber delight than some processed or fast foods that love to take up residence inside your upper thighs! The more you practice, the stronger and more toned you'll get and the more you'll be rewired to eat nourishing and delicious foods that your body can enjoy, use as fuel, and process efficiently.

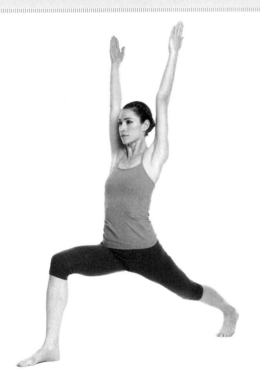

High Lunge Arms Up

Come into a low lunge. Press down through your feet and bring your torso up, aligning your shoulders above your hips. Inhale and lift your arms straight up. Relax your shoulders downward. Stay here for five long, deep breaths.

High Lunge Twist

From your high lunge with your arms still lifted, exhale and open your torso toward your right and open your arms. Sink your hips lower. Stay here for three long, deep breaths and come back to your high lunge.

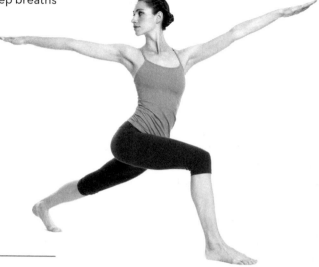

Warrior 3

From your high lunge, tip your torso forward so it's parallel to the ground. Shift your weight over your right leg and lift your back leg off the ground so it is parallel to the ground. Extend your arms straight out. Lengthen out through the top of your head and back through your back heel. Stay here for five long, deep breaths.

Do the routine on the other side.

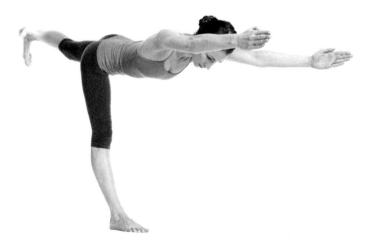

Killer Car Rides

Long car rides can be a total killer, but scrunched backs, hunched shoulders, tense minds, dulled energy, and tired eyes can all be remedied with a little yoga. And the most fun part about yoga for killer car rides is you can do the moves on your scheduled stops. All you need is just a little space, and you'll be all set to carry on your road trip with ease.

THE KILLER CAR RIDES YOGA CURE

A really fun way to reset your system while on a killer car ride is to do a lap around the car, or even the gas station or diner, on the next stop. (Keep an eye out for traffic, of course.) If you're traveling solo it may be safer to just do a lap around the car, and do a few of them, but with a group, a quick jog around the gas station or diner is good clean fun that will reboot your entire system. The following routine, minus the pigeon (unless you don't mind getting on the ground), can also be done whenever you pull the car over for a stop. The pigeon is a super great treat when you've reached your destination, though. Your hips will thank you!

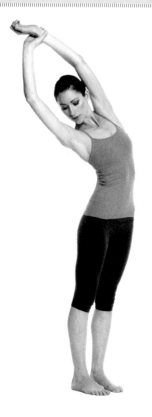

Standing Side Opener

Stand with your feet parallel to each other, shoulders aligned with your hips. Inhale and reach your arms out and up. Grab your left wrist with your right hand. Gently pull your left arm up with your right hand. Let your torso naturally arch over to your right side. Stay here for three long, deep breaths and then work the other side.

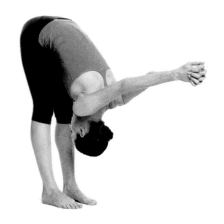

Standing Forward Bend Shoulder Opener

Stand comfortably with your feet a few inches apart. Inhale deeply. As you exhale, gently fold your torso forward over your legs. Interlace your hands behind you and let your arms fall over your back. If your hamstrings feel tense, bend your knees slightly and rest your belly on your thighs. Relax deeper into the pose with each exhale. Begin to lengthen your exhales a bit more than your inhales; this will encourage the body to open and the mind to settle. Stay here for five long, deep breaths.

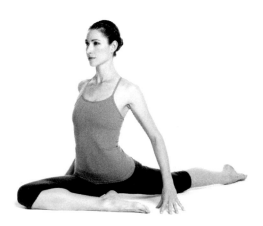

Pigeon

From your standing forward bend shoulder opener, release your fingertips to the ground, and step your left leg back to a low lunge. Move your right foot over toward your left hand and ease your knee down toward your right hand. If your hips don't reach the ground easily place a pillow or a blanket under them to bring the floor to you. Square your hips and shoulders to face forward. Stay here for three long, deep breaths. Inhale, crawl your fingertips back, and lift the chest. As you exhale, walk the fingertips forward and either rest on your forearms or make a pillow with your hands and rest your head. Stay here for ten long, deep breaths to release tension in the hips and mind.

Lack of Self-Esteem

A regular yoga practice is known to raise shrinking self-esteem levels and get you back to a nice, healthy confident range. Paying attention to how you feel in each pose, focusing on your breath, and keeping your attention on the internal instead of the external will help the worries, fears, and bad feelings about yourself fade away. The truth is, everything you need is right there inside, and always has been; you're wonderful as you are. Sometimes we forget, but yoga reminds us. We just have to get back on our feet and pay attention.

THE LACK OF SELF-ESTEEM YOGA CURE

The yoga cure for lack of self-esteem involves a lot of standing poses. When you make yourself stand, pay attention, breathe, and feel your strength, you are reminded that you are strong and capable of anything you set your intentions toward. The more you practice, the more your confidence builds. Watch out, you may feel like a superhero soon from all the yoga.

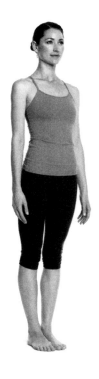

Standing

Stand at the top of your yoga mat. Feet are parallel and slightly apart, under your hip bones. Your hip bones aren't at the outside of your hips so make sure your feet aren't too far apart. You can check by placing two fists between your feet. That's about the width of your hip bones. Close your eyes and bring your attention to your breath. Lengthen and deepen your inhales and exhales and continue breathing at this nice slow pace for five full breaths. Gently open your eyes.

Warrior 2

Step your legs wide apart. Turn your right toes to face your front and your left toes slightly in so your hips and shoulders are facing your left. Open your arms straight out and away from your torso, right arm in front of you, and left arm behind you, palms down. Look over your front hand. Bend your right knee so your thigh is parallel to the ground. Stay here for ten long, deep breaths.

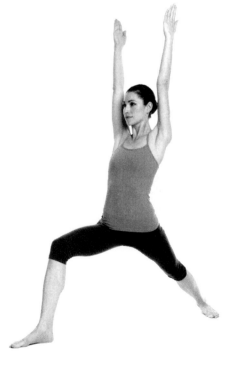

Warrior 2, Lift Arms Up

From your warrior 2, inhale and lift your hips and arms up. Exhale and lower back to Warrior 2. Repeat this same breath and movement pattern twice more.

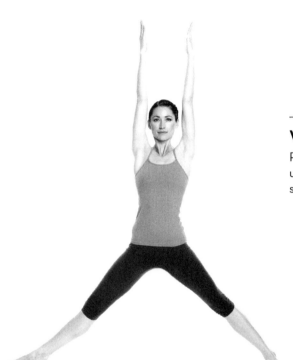

Warrior 1

From your warrior 2, bring your hips and shoulders to face forward. Adjust your feet so your arch of your back foot is in line with your front heel. Stay here for ten long, deep breaths and do the routine on the other side.

Laziness

Sometimes we get struck with a case of laziness. It can seemingly strike out of nowhere, or slowly build over time. Lounging around the house in vacation mode can be nice if we have some time off, but if you indulge yourself too much, loafing can become a habit, making it tough to follow your regular routine and attend to important tasks. A couple days of lazing around can easily lead to several more lazy days, then turn into habitual lazing around and get in the way of living a rich, full life. Sometimes you need a yoga cure to help you toss off the slippers and robe, throw yourself in the shower, get yourself together, and face the day ahead!

THE LAZINESS YOGA CURE

When loafing turns into laziness, a yoga cure can surely help. A simple spark of inspiration can get you back on track toward your optimal self. A case of laziness may or may not be clinically diagnosed, but for it to be cured, you need to actually get up and do something about it. Luckily, these yoga poses can help revitalize your entire system and inspire you to get back to your usual vibrant self. Try this routine daily until you are back on track.

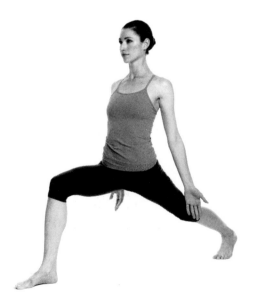

High Lunge Arms Down

Come into a low lunge. Press down through your feet to a standing lunge, reaching your arms behind you and bringing your shoulders in line with your hips. Relax your arms down by your sides, open your palms to face front, and sink your hips low. Stay here for three long, deep breaths.

High Lunge Arms Up

From your high lunge with arms down, inhale and lift your hips and arms up. As you exhale, sink back into your high lunge, arms down. Repeat this same breath and movement pattern twice more.

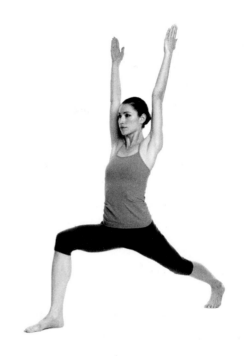

Warrior 2

From your high lunge, spin your back heel so your foot is planted on the ground, turn your right toes to face your front and your left toes slightly in so your hips and shoulders are facing your left. Open your arms straight out and away from your torso, right arm in front of you, and left arm behind you, palms down. Look over your front hand. Bend your right knee so your thigh is parallel to the ground. Stay here for ten long, deep breaths.

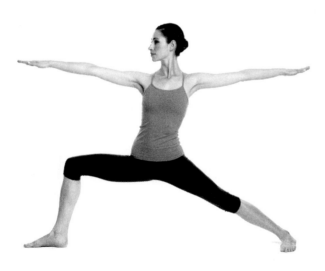

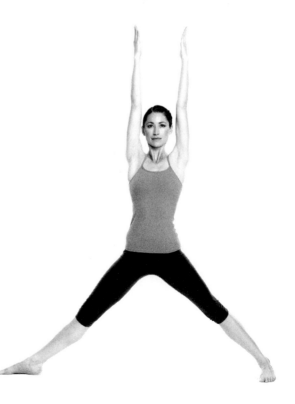

Warrior 2, Lift Arms Up

From your warrior 2, inhale and lift your hips and arms up. Exhale and lower back to warrior 2. Repeat this same breath and movement pattern twice more. Repeat the routine on the other side.

Migraine

The throbbing pain of an intense headache, sometimes accompanied by nausea, chills, fatigue, loss of appetite, numbness, vomiting, and sensitivity to light—no one wants to suffer through a migraine. Triggered by stress, certain foods, or some personal trigger, the attack begins in the various nerve pathways and affects blood flow to the brain and surrounding tissue. A regular yoga practice can help reduce the number of migraine episodes you experience, and help keep them from occurring in the first place. When they do strike, these simple poses and techniques can ease the pressure and tension in your head and make you more comfortable.

THE MIGRAINE YOGA CURE

Since a lot of migraines triggers have to do with stress, maintaining this simple routine at least three times a week will help. When a migraine does strike, this routine will ease pressure in your head, balance out your nervous system, and calm you down, encouraging the pain to move away.

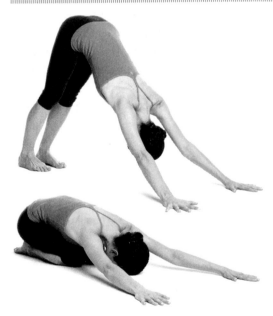

Down Dog

From all fours, tuck your toes, lift your hips, and press back into down dog. Reach your heels toward the ground. Relax your shoulders toward the ground and relax your head and neck. Stay here for five long, deep breaths.

Child's Pose

Gently come onto all fours. Relax your hips and sit back on your heels. Rest your forehead on the ground and breathe deeply into your back. Stay here for five long, deep breaths.

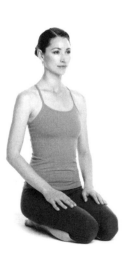

Temple Massage

From your child's pose, sit up on your heels. Press your index fingers into the center of your eyebrows, then trace an arch up your forehead and out to the sides of your temples, pressing evenly as you go. Repeat this movement three more times.

Monkey Mind

"Monkey mind" is yoga slang for someone whose mind is all over the place, like a monkey, one second focused on a banana, the other jumping from place to place, the next, back to the banana—we've all been there. Ever start a project as simple as writing an e-mail, stop mid-sentence, go and browse the fridge, look through a pile of mail, browse a magazine, and remember the e-mail after all of that? A hectic lifestyle that goes unmanaged can add to the severity of monkey mind. You are what you practice, and there is a way to get your mind focused and under control no matter how clear or cluttered your calendar is. If you practice racing to work, racing to appointments, and never actually being in the present moment, monkey mind will catch you. The good news is you can rid your mind of its monkey business with these simple techniques practiced at least three times a week.

THE MONKEY MIND YOGA CURE

The yoga cure for monkey mind is to observe your little monkey. Observation without judgment allows us to take a slight step back from our own selves and see what is really going on in there. When we gain space and perspective, the monkey mind simply dissolves and we are left clear and focused. When you observe a racing, scattered mind, it has no choice but to settle (kind of like a little kid whose mom is staring at him as he's about to do something naughty). It's the trick of distraction. Distractions are only distracting if you let them be. If you stare them in the eye, they go away, just like tension. When you breathe into tension, it eventually dissolves. When you observe monkey mind, the monkey sits down and listens.

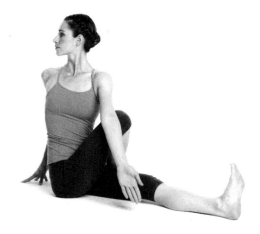

Seated Spine Twist

Sit up tall and extend both legs out in front of you. Hug your right knee in toward your chest and place your right foot on the ground close to your body, outside your left leg. Inhale your left arm up and cross it over your right leg. Press your right fingertips behind your hips. Inhale and sit up tall. Exhale and twist your torso further to the right. Repeat this same breath and movement pattern twice more and then do the other side.

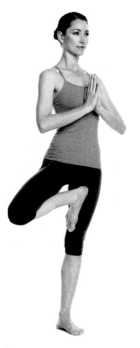

Tree, Hands in Prayer

Shift your weight onto your left leg. Draw your right knee into your chest, grab your ankle, and press the bottom of your right foot onto your left thigh. If you feel wobbly keep your hand on your ankle while it's pressed into your thigh. If you're finding your balance really easily, reach your arms straight up or press your palms together in front of your chest. If this is challenging in an overwhelming way, place your toes on the ground and rest your foot onto your ankle. Press your palms together in front of your chest. Stay here for ten long, deep breaths. Come back to standing for ten long, deep breaths and try the same thing on the other side.

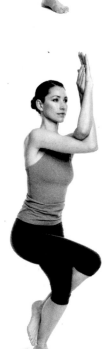

Eagle

Hug your right knee into your chest. Bend your left knee and cross your right leg around your left leg, hooking your right foot on either side of your left leg. Wrap your right arm under your left arm. Sit down as much as you lift up through the arms to stay on balance. Stay here for five long, deep breaths. Unwind and do the same thing on the other side.

Office Body

Are you suffering from slumped shoulders, burning eyes, achy joints, and cramped muscles from spending most of your time chained to a desk? Pretty much anyone who has a job these days is spending way too many hours at the computer, sitting in meetings, and rushing everywhere. Working in our modern age leaves us with a super tight, cramped, and tense body, impossibly tight hips, hunched shoulders, painful wrists, burning eyes, and of course a big heap of anxiety. Fortunately, a regular yoga practice can combat these symptoms, so you can get through your workday without wrecking your body.

THE OFFICE BODY YOGA CURE

This routine is designed to release tension in your shoulders, hips, and hamstrings, and open up the spine. If you practice every day, the tension that builds while you're at your desk won't have a fighting chance against all your Zen efforts. Do this routine in the morning before work and at night when you come home to release all the tension of office body.

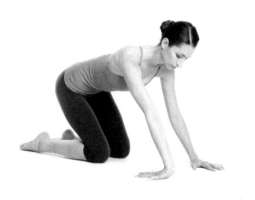

Hands and Knees Wrist Release

Move onto your hands and knees. Make sure your wrists are under your shoulders and your knees are under your hips. Keep your spine nice and neutral. Spread your fingers wide. Turn your right hand as far to the right as it will go, so the heel of your hand is facing forward and your fingers are facing your body. Roll your body around slightly, getting the stretch into different areas of your wrist. Breathe into any tight areas. Stay with this for five long, deep breaths and then do the other side.

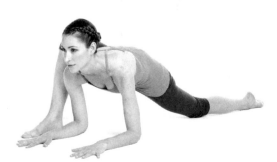

Lizard

From your last pose go into a low lunge, with your right leg forward. Move your right foot over toward your right hand, keeping your toes pointing forward. Lower your back knee down to the ground. If your hips feel super tight, stay here and breathe. If your body allows you more room to work within this pose, gently lower your forearms to the ground. Stay here for ten long, deep breaths.

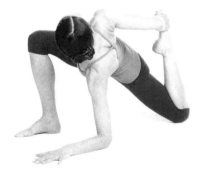

Lizard Twist with Ankle Hold

From your lizard, if there is room in your body without feeling tense, bend your back (left) knee, spin your torso toward your right (in the direction of your front leg), and grab your left foot with your right hand. Gently pull your foot in toward your hips. Stay here for three long, deep breaths and repeat on the other side beginning with the lizard pose.

Office Mind

Now that we've covered office body, we have the mind to take into consideration. When your brain feels like it's bursting from overflowing e-mails, endless meetings, spreadsheets, and to-do lists, you are having an attack of office mind! When your mind gets frazzled at the office, you might be going through the motions of your work, but the clarity and focus is out the window, and forget about any joy and ease. Culprits are dry and irritated eyes from staring at a computer screen, deadline-induced anxieties, office politics, a lack of work/life balance, and whatever other challenges you deal with at your workplace. They all add up quickly to a cranky, stuck state of being, or office mind. Not good. Fortunately, yoga can help.

THE OFFICE MIND YOGA CURE

Bringing a little more "you time" into your workdays will help a ton, by calming anxiety, releasing tension in the eyes, and relaxing your entire body so when new tension tries to enter, it rolls right off you. Do this routine in the morning before work and when you get home. If you can squeeze it in at midday, all the better.

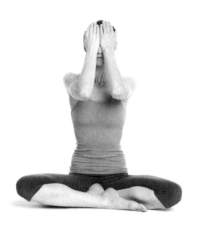

Calm Eyes

Sit up comfortably, nice and tall. Rub the palms of your hands together pretty quickly to get a good amount of heat going. Close your eyes and gently press the heels of your hands into your eyelids. Rest your fingers against your forehead. Stay here for three long, deep breaths and gently relax your hands to rest on your thighs.

Four-Count Breathing

From your seated position take in a big inhale through your nose, and exhale all the air out through your mouth. Inhale through your nose on a slow count to four. At the top hold your breath in for another slow count of four. Then exhale through your nose for another slow count of four. Repeat this breathing pattern ten times.

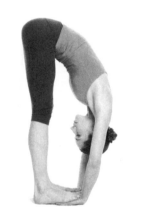

Standing Forward Bend, Step on Hands

Stand up tall with your shoulders aligned with your hips. Bend your knees slightly and slowly roll down your spine, head first, until your torso is gently hanging over your legs. Step on the palms of your hands so that the tops of your hands are on the ground, toes on the insides of your wrists. Relax your head and neck. Stay here for ten long, deep breaths.

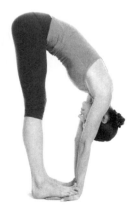

Standing Forward Bend, Step on Palms

From your standing forward bend, step on hands, gently remove your hands from under your feet. Turn your hands outward and step on the tops of your hands (palms on the ground) so your toes are touching your wrists. Relax your head and neck. Stay here for ten long, deep breaths.

Overweight/Obesity

A regular yoga practice has been shown time after time to bring people to a healthy weight when diets and other forms of exercise have failed them. Why? Because yoga is a sustainable, transformative practice that teaches us how to pay attention. Simply put, practicing yoga makes people mindful of what and how they eat, and that can help prevent the dread phenomenon of middle-age spread in normal-weight people. In addition, it may promote weight loss in those who are overweight. We get sensitive to the needs of our bodies and as a result our desires and cravings naturally shift toward foods that are nourishing rather than destructive. The more we practice, the more mindfulness settles into our bodies and our lives and taking care of ourselves in every way becomes second nature.

REAL-LIFE CURES: Durk's Drastic Weight Loss

Durk, a six-foot-four-inch 250-plus-pound guy started yoga for fitness and stress reduction purposes, and also as a fun way to spend time with his girlfriend. After a few classes this jovial guy developed a desire to prepare more of his meals at home; he wanted a lot of veggies and no longer craved fried foods and lots of meats, which were a big part of his previous diet. His newfound eating habits, coupled with yoga practice three to four times a week, helped Durk drop over forty pounds in four months. His high blood pressure has lowered to a healthy number, and he has even more energy and excitement for life than he did before. And to top it off he can now get his legs up over his heart in a shoulder stand, a tricky pose for heavier people because it involves lifting your hips over your head, and a large torso can get in the way. Shoulder stand is a fantastic pose that corrects a lot of imbalances in the body, including regulating the thyroid gland, which is extremely helpful when on a path toward weight loss. Every day gets more exciting for Durk. With every class he feels easier and lighter in his body and mind. Durk always has a huge smile on his face.

The Overweight/Obesity Yoga Cure

When beginning yoga with the goal of losing weight, start slow. There is no need to push or force anything or even begin with a commitment to a seven-day-a-week practice. Prepare yourself to be open; allow your body and mind space to begin a new path toward lasting, radiant health. Start practicing once a week for a few weeks to get in the yoga zone, and after a few weeks feel free to step it up to three or four times a week or more, depending on how you feel. Soon, you'll be hooked on feeling great with the yoga that you'll be practicing every day.

Meditation is important and so beneficial when it comes to weight loss. Try to set a regular time for meditation practice first thing in the morning. You can even meditate right from your bed. Try this routine three to four times a week. Do the meditation daily.

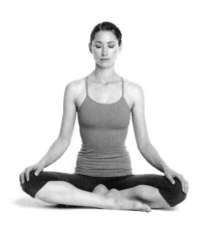

Seated Meditation

Sit up nice and tall, however you can sit most comfortably. Relax your shoulders, so that they are away from your ears. Rest your palms on your thighs (face up or face down, whichever is most comfortable for you) and close your eyes. Start to rest your attention on your breath. Watch your inhales come and exhales go. Settle your mind in the space between. Begin to lengthen and deepen your inhales and exhales, setting a slow, easy pace of breathing. If a thought starts to enter your mind, simply observe it like a cloud passing by. Let the thought pass and come back to your breath. Continue observing your breath for three to five minutes. A stopwatch could come in handy, or you could simply feel it out and see how much time has actually passed when you open your eyes. Either way is useful.

Do this practice for at least five minutes in the morning, five minutes during some part of your day, whether at work, during a commute (in a train, bus, or cab, not if you're driving), and before bed at night. A regular meditation practice will ease your mind and help you relax your body. Also fantastic for dealing with cravings, urges, and the tendency to binge, purge, eat out of anxiety, or eat rushed. Meditation sensitizes your entire system so you will begin to enjoy your food more. Your sense of taste, touch, and smell will actually begin to heighten. Enjoy the journey!

Now we'll practice a moving meditation with some sun salutations. Let the breath be the only "yoga pose" on which you focus. Your body will move into the poses naturally; let it follow your breath. If you notice your body tensing, that's good because it means you're paying attention; just simply guide your attention back to your breath. A lot of weight loss is about relaxation, about finding the ease in effort, both on and off the mat. Finding ease on the mat will help you find it in life, and it will change the way you relate to eating.

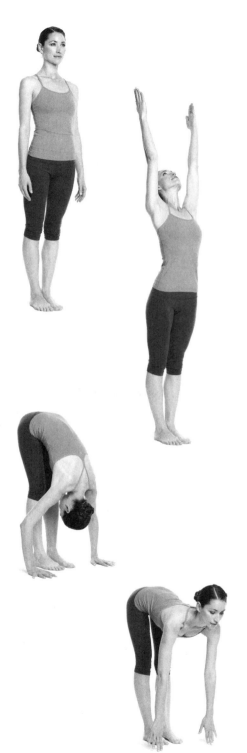

SUN SALUTATIONS

Sun Salutations warm up, lengthen, and strengthen your entire body and calm your mind simultaneously.

Standing

Stand at the top of your yoga mat. Feet are parallel and slightly apart, under your hip bones. Your hip bones aren't at the outside of your hips so make sure your feet aren't too far apart. You can check by placing two fists between your feet. That's about the width of your hip bones. Close your eyes and bring your attention to your breath. Lengthen and deepen your inhales and exhales and continue breathing at this nice slow pace for five full breaths. Gently open your eyes.

Standing Arm Reach

Inhale and lift your arms out to your sides and up, filling up all the space with your breath and your movement. Relax your tailbone and lift your chest. Keep your shoulders relaxed down your back and look up while keeping your face and the skin of your forehead relaxed.

Standing Forward Bend

Exhale and bend your trunk forward over your legs. Let your head and neck relax and hang heavy. If your hamstrings feel tight, keep a slight bend in your knees to give them some more space to relax and open. Press your fingertips on the ground.

Standing Forward Bend with Arch

Inhale, look forward, and lengthen out your back, so that it's horizontal. Let your fingertips graze the ground. If that's too much stress on your hamstrings, press your hands lightly into your shins to get a nice length in your spine.

Plank

Press your palms firmly into the ground and step your feet back to plank. Make sure your wrists are under your shoulders and your knees are under your hips. Spread your fingers wide. Tuck your toes under and straighten your legs and arms, bringing your body into a straight line from the top of your head through the bottoms of your heels. Keep your stomach strong and lift the front of your thighs up. Stay here for five long, deep breaths. If this is too intense gently lower your knees to the floor. Always make sure you can breathe easily during this pose.

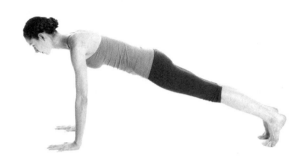

Plank Push-Up

Bend your elbows straight back and lower your body halfway down in one straight line until your upper arms are parallel to the ground. If a half push-up is too intense you can either lower your knees so they're touching the ground, and then bend your elbows to lower halfway, or slowly lower all the way down to your belly by bending your elbows straight back.

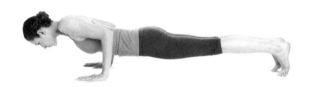

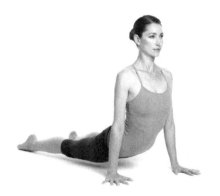

Up Dog

Lower your knees gently to the ground. Roll your shoulders down your back and lift your chest through your arms with a big inhale. Straighten your arms as much as feels comfortable, keeping your shoulders down back. If you straighten your arms and your back feels pinched, bend the elbows and continue to lift your chest through your arms until you feel good. Sway your torso a little from side to side if that feels good. Keep your body easy, never forced or tense.

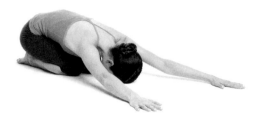

Child's Pose

Gently come onto all fours. Relax your hips and sit back on your heels. Rest your forehead on the ground and breathe deeply into your back. Stay here for five long, deep breaths.

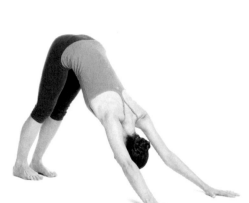

Down Dog

When you are ready, spread your fingers wide, lift your hips, tuck your toes, and press back into down dog. Reach your heels down toward the ground, relax your shoulders toward the ground, and relax your neck. Gently sway from side to side. Experiment on your own with easy movements to match your easy breath, to help open up the body and calm the mind. Stay in down dog for five long, deep breaths.

Then slowly walk your feet up to your hands, back to your standing forward bend. Keeping your head and neck heavy roll up to standing, one vertebra at a time. Once you reach the top, inhale your arms out and up, filling up all the space with all of you, and you'll be back where we started. Repeat five times or more to create some heat in the body and ease of mind.

Plank

Get on all fours. Make sure your wrists are under your shoulders and your knees are under your hips. Spread your fingers wide, tuck your toes under, and straighten your legs and arms, bringing your body into a straight line from the top of your head through the bottoms of your heels. Keep your stomach nice and strong and lift the front of your thighs up. If this is too intense feel free to gently lower your knees to the floor. Always make sure you can breathe easily during this pose.

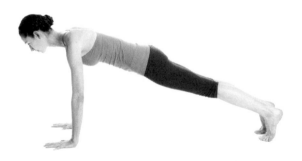

We're going to stay here for a while. This simple pose can teach us that we are strong enough to hold our own bodies up. Our mind may try to tell us otherwise. If your mind starts to tense, remember that your arms will not fall off and your body will be energized when this is finished, and come back to your breath. Stay in your plank pose for ten long, deep breaths. Find the ease in the effort. Allowing your body to stay in plank this way will ease anxiety that is related to all sorts of things, including anxious eating. It will also strengthen the body from the inside out, toning your shoulders, thighs, and your entire abdominal region. The most important benefit is learning how to be easy during challenging circumstances. If you need a break, rest in child's pose, but come back into the plank. And do it every day too! It gets way easier with practice. I promise!

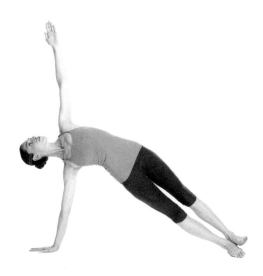

Side Plank

From your plank, lift your hips, press down with your right hand, roll to the outside edge of your right foot. Stack the left foot on top of the right. Open your entire body to your left side. Keep the hips lifted, expand through the chest, extend your left arm and fingers straight up and turn your gaze toward your left fingers. You can either stay here, or lower the right knee down to the ground. When your breathing moves away from long and deep toward short and fast, it's a good idea to back off the pose. Forcing and pushing your body only leads to tension and injury. Stay here for three long, deep breaths, roll through your plank pose, and try the other side.

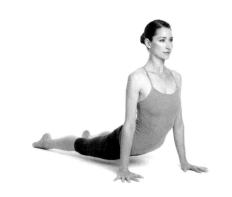

Up Dog

Lower your knees gently to the ground. Roll your shoulders away from your ears and lift your chest through your arms with a big inhale. Straighten your arms as much as feels comfortable keeping your shoulders down and back. If your back feels okay (no pain at all), press down through the tops of your feet and straighten your knees. Stay here for two long, deep inhales and exhales.

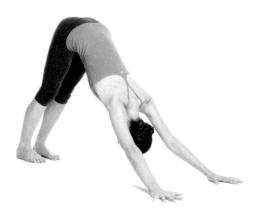

Down Dog

On an exhale tuck your toes reach your hips back and up and your heels down toward the ground, and press back into your down dog. Stay here for five long, deep breaths.

You can repeat this routine from down dog by rolling into plank, moving into side plank on one side, and then the other, sinking through up dog, and lifting back to down dog. Practicing with the eyes closed really draws the attention inward, and also challenges your body awareness and balance, which is fun!

Party Pooper

Yoga reminds us that we can be fun, even if we've forgotten, or even lost that part of ourselves along the way by being serious in life. Yoga has a way of bringing the joy back to you. Feel it overflow as you go from party pooper to life of the party. When in life do we get a chance to actually fall down and have it be not only all right, but encouraged?

Most of us have gotten caught up in our self image, at least at some point, if not all the time. "I am a serious person. I do serious work. I think serious things and have serious things to say." It's useful if we can learn to be at ease with ourselves, to give ourselves a break from the grown-up at your shoulder and lighten up. You can get all the serious work you need to accomplish in your life done and still have a lot of fun. There is no rule that you have to have a frown on your face and be stern to be taken seriously.

Anyone who has attempted a handstand or any other balance pose has probably taken quite a few topples, and how can you not find the fun in that?

REAL-LIFE CURES: Tara's Smiles for Miles

I was driving to the airport in Los Angeles and having a "serious moment." I was reflecting on yoga, thinking about the studio in New York, and, without realizing it, taking myself way too seriously. At a stoplight, a car pulled up next to me and through our rolled-down windows the driver looked over to me and said, "Smile, you should lighten up."

Granted, it was an odd thing for me at the time. My instinct was to roll up the window, lock the doors, and gun the light. I was definitely taken off guard, mostly because I was so deeply into my serious moment that I would never have considered a smile, but he was right. I did smile, just a little, and it worked. I immediately felt better and was taken out of my stuck moment. You never know where you are going to find your yoga teachers! They might not always be sitting in the front of a yoga class.

THE PARTY POOPER YOGA CURE

The cure for a party pooper is to shift balance, change perspective, turn the moment upside down, and have fun while you're at it. If we practice yoga in super-serious mode we are missing its joy. Finding, living, and sharing joy is what yoga (like life) is all about. Joy is in you whether you deny it or embrace it. Ninety-three-year-young yoga master Tao Porchon-Lynch, my good friend, always says that nature is her encyclopedia. It is always recycling itself, finding and expressing the joy of life with ease. Tao teaches us to remember that we are nature. Sometimes we have to remind ourselves to find the ease and then get back to the joy and fun of life that is the natural essence of our existence and the essence of yoga.

Fair warning: this routine is designed to show you a good time. Your first step is to be ready to have fun, or at least open to the possibility of lightening your load just a bit. Try this routine a couple times a week to start, and soon you may be having such a ball that you will want to do it every day!

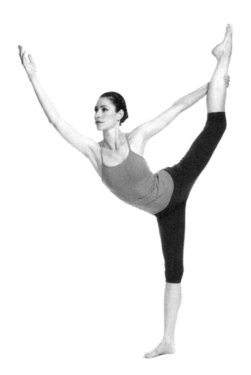

Dancer

Stand up straight, feet a few inches apart and parallel. Stack your shoulders so that they are aligned with the top of your hips. Close your eyes. Take a big inhale through your nose. Exhale out through your mouth.

Shift your weight onto your right leg. Bend your left knee and grab hold of the inside of your left calf with your left hand. Find something in front of you to focus on. Take two long, deep inhales and exhales while standing on the one foot. Begin to press your left foot into your left hand. The pressure of the foot into the hand will open up the back. Only press as much as you can easily, without a lot of resistance. Reach your right arm straight up.

Don't worry about the shape of the pose. Keep your breath long, deep, and relaxed and allow your body to move where it can with ease. Now if you haven't already done so, simply tip yourself over and topple out of the pose. It's good for you. Try the pose a few times playing with your balance. Don't forget to smile and have fun.

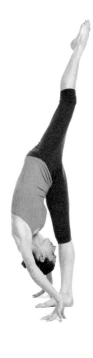

Standing Split

Bring both hands to the floor and touch your fingertips to the ground right under your shoulders. Allow the left leg and hip to open and release, as you lift it up behind you. Walk your fingertips back so they are in line with your toes. Release your head and neck toward the standing leg. Take three long, deep breaths, favoring the exhales a bit more than the inhales. Repeat on the other side . . . and again feel free to fall if you need to here.

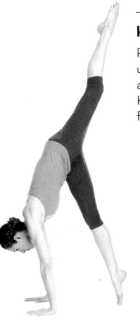

Handstand Rocks

From your standing split press your palms firmly on the ground under your shoulders. Straighten your arms. Keep the left leg lifted and rock forward and back, trying to get your hips over shoulders. Keep breathing through the entire movement. Inhale as you rock forward and exhale as you release.

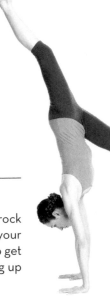

Handstand L Shape

See if the bottom foot wants to leave the ground as you rock forward. Rest your gaze between your hands. Lift up in your belly as you rock forward to give yourself an extra boost to get some air. Try little hops on that right leg and lift the left leg up so your legs will be in the shape of the letter L.

Handstand

If you are finding some balance in your handstand L shape bring the legs together at the top. Keep your arms strong and steady and your gaze focused but soft on the ground between your hands. There are a bunch of fun ways to topple out of a handstand. You can cartwheel out of it, flip your body into a backbend, walk the hands a bit till you can bring the feet back to the ground, or make up your own way. Remember, yoga is experiential. It's your experience.

Make sure to breathe through the routine and repeat it on the other side, too!

PMS and Cramps

A monthly ordeal for many, PMS and cramps can cause symptoms ranging from pain and discomfort to increased irritability, sensitivity, and aggressiveness. The list is slightly different for each person. Here are some simple yoga poses that can help you deal with the discomfort, so you no longer have to put up with it every month.

THE PMS AND CRAMPS YOGA CURE

This routine is designed to calm the body, relieve the pressure and pain of cramps, reduce anxiety, and level the over-the-top emotions that can go along with your monthly cycle. When practiced regularly, this routine can reduce these uncomfortable symptoms over time.

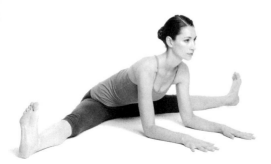

Child's Pose Twist

Come into a child's pose. Reach your hips to your heels, relax your forehead on the ground, and extend your arms out in front of you. Thread your left arm under your right arm so your whole left shoulder and the left side of your face are resting on the ground. Stay here for five long, deep breaths and then do the same on the other side.

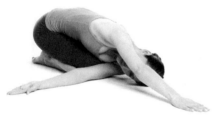

Seated, Both Legs Straight Forward Bend (blanket on lap)

Roll up a blanket. Sit down with your legs straight in front of you. Place the blanket on your upper thighs. Gently fold your torso over the blanket. Stay here for ten long, deep breaths.

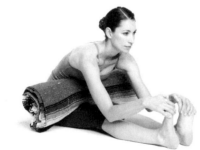

Seated Wide Leg Straddle

Sit up tall and open your legs to the sides until you feel a little tension, but not so much that it is uncomfortable. Walk your hands forward between your legs and keep your torso long. Stay here for ten long, deep breaths, favoring the exhales a bit more than the inhales to encourage tension to release.

Pregnancy Discomfort

Continuing or beginning a regular yoga practice during pregnancy can be a fantastic way to reduce anxiety about labor and everything else that goes along with bringing a life onto the planet. It can also strengthen the body, release tension in the muscles, create a good range of motion, and focus the mind. If you are brand new to yoga, it's probably not a terrific idea to start a hard-core regimen during pregnancy, but there are a variety of prenatal yoga poses and techniques that are gentle and still very effective that can help you breeze through your pregnancy, and also help with your upcoming labor.

A study conducted by the Vivekananda Yoga Research Foundation in India indicates that a daily yoga and meditation practice during pregnancy seems to improve birth weight and reduce prematurity and overall medical complications for newborns. "A consistent yoga practice can produce a healthier maternal environment for pregnancy and a significantly gentler and more harmonious birthing experience for both mother and child," said Dr. Sejal Shah, one of the researchers who conducted the study.

Easy, gentle yoga stimulates the reproductive organs to ensure a relatively easy childbirth, ensures optimum blood supply and nutrients to the developing fetus, enhances correct posture, establishes a balance between the sympathetic and parasympathetic nervous systems, improves blood circulation, tones the muscles of the spine, abdomen, and pelvis (helping to support the added weight of the uterus), and prevents common ailments such as backache, leg cramps, breathlessness, and edema in the feet. These are all good things for a woman whose body is working hard throughout pregnancy.

REAL-LIFE CURES: Simone's Yoga Switch

Simone had been a gym junkie for years until she got pregnant with her firstborn child, a baby girl. She had always known of the benefits of yoga but wanted to do cardio and weights to get more of a "workout." But early in her pregnancy, Simone found herself wandering into a prenatal group class and found not only the stress reduction she was looking for, but also a fantastic way to work out the body and the mind at the same time. Now, after the birth of her little one, Simone is a yoga regular, using it as her primary stress reducer as well as her workout regimen.

The Pregnancy Discomfort Yoga Cure

There are a few things to consider when beginning or continuing a yoga practice during pregnancy. Paying attention to how you are feeling is extremely important. A regular yoga practice will sensitize you so you know when things are a little off or don't feel quite right. Listen to your instincts. It's commonly agreed that in the first trimester all twists should be avoided. Many instructors steer away from inversions such as headstands and handstands, especially if the person is new to them. Pay attention to your body. Talk to your doctor. And talk to other pregnant women if you have the chance. The sense of community and support found in prenatal yoga classes can be even more beneficial than the yoga poses. If you are taking a regular yoga class, one not specified as prenatal, let your instructor know what month you are in so together you can adjust your routine as needed. Also, remember to have fun, enjoy the breath, and enjoy your changing body. Yoga can help you embrace the changes with ease and a sense of adventure.

This routine can be done in any phase of pregnancy and is designed to ease the mind and release tension in the hips and hamstrings. Do this as often as makes you feel comfortable. First thing in the morning and last thing at night is a great start.

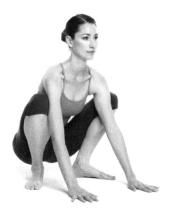

Squat

Stand tall with your feet shoulder width apart. Turn your toes out to the sides, and your heels in. Sink your hips down toward the ground. If your heels don't reach the ground bring a blanket to put under them for extra support. Place your hands on the ground in front of you for support.

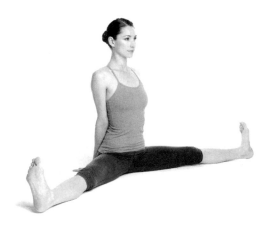

Wide Leg Straddle (upright)

Sit on the floor or a mat and open your legs out to the sides. Open them only as far as you can without tension. Press your fingertips into the floor behind your hips and lift your chest up. Flex your feet and reach through your heels. Stay here for three long, deep breaths.

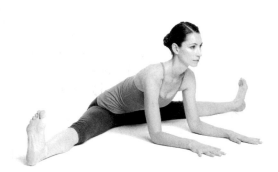

Wide Leg Straddle (lowered torso)

If you feel like you have more room to work within this pose, walk your hands out in front of you, keeping your back nice and long. Only go as far as you can while feeling just a bit of tension, but enough that you can breathe into the position easily. Stay here for ten long, deep breaths.

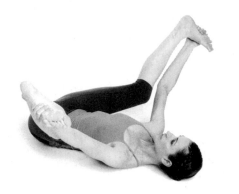

Happy Baby

Lie down on your back. Draw your knees into your chest. Grab the outsides of your feet with your hands so the bottoms of your feet point straight up. Gently pull your knees down toward the ground outside your torso using the strength of your arms. If it feels good rock carefully from side to side to open your back and hips even more. Stay here for ten long, deep breaths.

Procrastination

Need to get something done but keep putting it off until the last possible minute? We've all experienced procrastination at some point in our lives. It can be accompanied by denial, followed by anxiety, frustration, and downright panic when we get right up to our deadline. Often we simply lack the tools to pace ourselves or set a schedule that would lead us to accomplish our tasks on time. When something is overwhelming, we may ignore it until the last minute, sending ourselves into a frenzy. We need to be prepared so we can spot it and do something about it. Yoga can help by releasing excess tension in the mind that may be blocking those creative juices. Yoga will also build focus so you can concentrate without distraction on the task at hand. Often when we have a task ahead of us that we feel anxious about completing, we stop in the middle before we complete it. When we feel inspired, we have the energy and desire to continue with the tasks we set out to accomplish and do them with ease and focus. This routine is designed to ignite, or possibly rekindle, your desire to dive right into your projects and maintain focus throughout until completion.

THE PROCRASTINATION YOGA CURE

The best way to alleviate procrastination is to get inspired. When you have lasting inspiration any project, deadline, or drawer that needs cleaning will get the focused attention it needs without the stress.

So without further anticipation, or procrastination, let's get right to the yoga. This routine is designed to invigorate your entire body and ease tension in the mind. Stay with the breath and have fun! Do this routine at least three times a week to get yourself back on track.

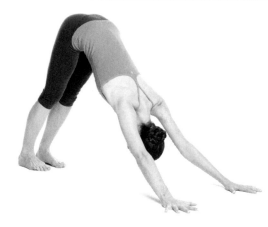

Down Dog

From all fours, tuck your toes, lift your hips, and press back into down dog. Reach your heels toward the ground. Relax your shoulders toward the ground and relax your head and neck. Stay here for five long, deep breaths.

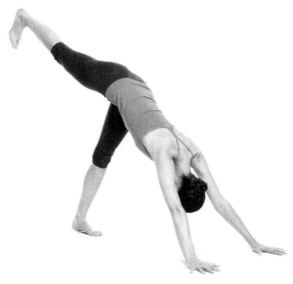

Down Dog Split

From your down dog, inhale and lift your right leg straight up. Flex your foot and reach through the heel as if you are helping to hold up a wall with your foot. Square the hips so the toes of your right foot are pointing down and lift up from the back of the upper thigh. Continue to press through both arms evenly as you extend out through the leg.

Pigeon

As you exhale, draw your right knee in toward your forehead and guide the foot to rest behind your left hand and rest your knee on the ground by your right hand, so your shin is working toward parallel to the front of your mat. Square your hips and shoulders to face forward. Stay here for three long, deep breaths. Inhale, crawl your fingertips back, and lift your chest. As you exhale, walk the fingertips forward and either rest on your forearms or make a pillow with your hands and rest your head. Stay here for ten long, deep breaths to release tension in your hips, and your mind.

When you are ready to come up, slowly walk your fingertips back by your hips and stack your shoulders above your hips. Press your palms down under your shoulders and make your way back to down dog.

Make sure to breathe through the routine and repeat it on the other side, too!

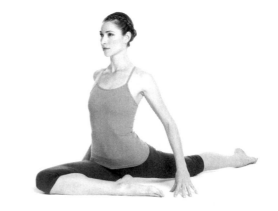

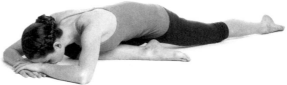

Runners' Aches

If you are a runner, you should pick up a yoga mat on your next run and get right down to practicing regularly. Along with the benefits of improved flexibility, you'll also gain an improved range of motion in the rest of your body, which can make you faster and more efficient. Injury prevention is a superb benefit of yoga. The improved lung capacity you'll gain with yoga will also give you an advantage over competitors. When it comes to preventing or recovering from injuries, as well as dealing with daily aches and pains from running, yoga can be a great therapy for your body and a de-stressor for the mind.

THE RUNNERS' ACHES YOGA CURE

This routine is designed to open the chest and spine to increase lung capacity and mobility in the torso, and ease soreness in the upper body. It also works to release tension in the big muscle groups of the hips and hamstrings.

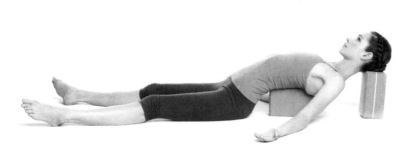

Supported Bridge with 2 Blocks

Have two blocks handy. Place one block on the ground lengthwise. Sit down in front of the block. Keeping your hips on the ground, lie your spine down along the block. Place the other block under your head. Relax your legs out in front of you and stay here for twenty long, deep breaths.

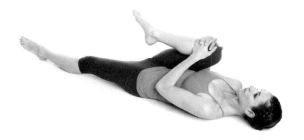

Reclining Single Knee Hug

Gently bring yourself off the block and lie back down on your back. Hug your right knee into your chest. With each exhale, draw your knee closer toward your right shoulder. Stay here for five long, deep breaths.

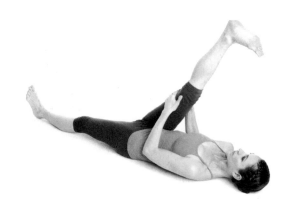

Reclining Hamstring Release

Extend your right leg upward. Grab behind your calf, your knee, or your hamstring, wherever you can grab easily and comfortably. Stay here for ten long, deep breaths. Try not to pull the leg closer toward you, but instead allow your exhales to release tension and naturally move your leg closer when more space opens up.

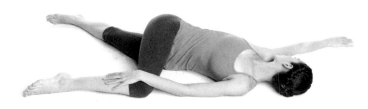

Relining Single Knee Hug Twist

Bend your knee back into your chest. Open your arms out to the sides and cross your right leg over toward your left. Stay here for ten long, deep breaths.

Do the routine on the other side beginning with the reclining knee hug.

Saggy Booty

Yes, the benefits of yoga run deep and include lowering high blood pressure, decreasing the risk of diabetes, and reducing anxiety, but let's be honest, yoga has some pretty fantastic benefits for your booty as well. And these would be a shame to ignore. Your yoga practice is a one-stop shop for a radiantly healthy body from the inside out—the "out" being a sweet reward.

THE SAGGY BOOTY YOGA CURE

The following yoga poses are the best booty shapers on the market, which might be one of the best-kept secrets of the fitness industry. You can do all the squats and lunges you want at the gym, but doing these yoga poses regularly will get right to that burn you're looking for and will carve out that lifted, toned shape you'll be proud to show off when you sashay across the room. So you might as well treat it well and tone it up! While you are twisting, holding, and balancing your way through the poses, you are carving out an uplifted, toned, long, lean, and strong lower half. The upper half of your body is getting toned also, but we'll get to that in a bit.

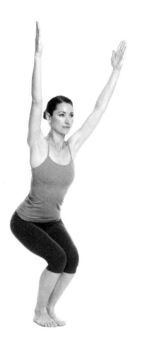

Chair

Stand up tall with your feet under your hips and parallel to each other. Inhale and sink your hips low. Reach your arms up overhead. Relax your shoulders down toward your back. Relax the area in front of your ribs and lengthen your spine. Stay here for ten long, deep breaths.

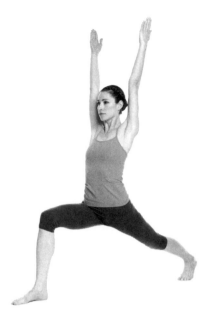

High Lunge

From your chair, gently fold your torso over your legs. Press your fingertips into the ground and step your left leg back to a low lunge. Press down through your feet and bring your torso up, aligning your shoulders above your hips. Inhale and lift your arms straight up. Relax your shoulders down toward your back. Stay here for five long, deep breaths.

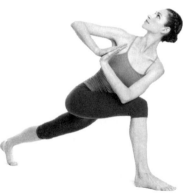

High Lunge with Prayer Twist

From your high lunge, press your palms together in front of your chest. Inhale and lift your chest and your palms. As you exhale twist toward your front leg. Press your left elbow into the outside of your front thigh. Press down firmly through your top hand into your bottom hand to turn your torso further to the side. Lift your belly away from your top thigh. Reach out evenly through the top of your head and out through your back heel. Stay here for five long, deep breaths.

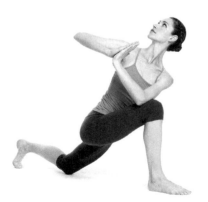

High Lunge with Prayer Twist (back knee down)

If it's tricky to find the balance in your high lunge with prayer twist, gently lower your back knee down and continue the twist. Stay here for five long, deep breaths.

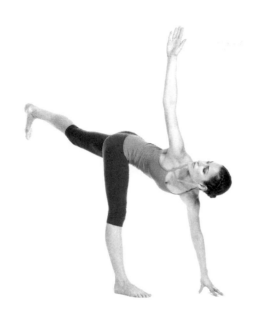

Twisted Half Moon

From the previous pose, open up your arms and press your left fingertips into the ground inside of your front foot, directly under your left shoulder. Shift your weight onto your right leg and lift your back leg up so it is parallel to the ground, keeping your hips square. Move your left fingertips forward so they stay pressed into the ground under your left shoulder. Open your torso to the right and lengthen your right arm up over your right shoulder. Stay here for three long, deep breaths.

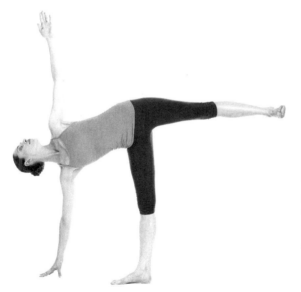

Half Moon

From your half-moon twist, press your right fingertips into the ground under your right shoulder. Roll your left hip so that it aligns on top of your right and your torso faces left. Lift your left arm up over your left shoulder and look up toward your left hand. Stay here for three long, deep breaths.

Perform the routine on the other side, beginning with chair pose.

Saggy Pecs

While we are busy getting healthy and happy from the inside out, an amazing side effect happens naturally with regular practice: our bodies take the shape that they are meant to—toned, strong, and lean. A droopy body is a result of sedentary muscles, and can be remedied. Saggy pecs can be perked right up with some simple yoga poses targeted to fire up and build the muscles of the chest and shoulders. The result will leave you with perky pecs and better posture.

THE SAGGY PECS YOGA CURE

The cure for saggy pecs is simply to begin strengthening the upper body with consistent practice. The good news is that there are a few fantastic poses that will target the pecs so you will build a strong, lean, firm, and lifted upper body. Regular practice is essential to maintain strength and muscle tone, so even though you will feel the burn with this routine after doing it once, keep doing it every day for lasting results.

Forearm Plank

Bring yourself to all fours. Lower your forearms to the ground so they are parallel to each other. Lengthen your legs straight behind you, tuck your toes, and straighten your legs. Your body should be in one long, straight line from the top of your head to your heels.

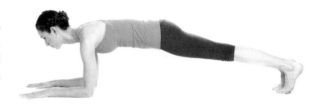

Plank

Press into your palms, straighten your arms, and come into a plank. Make sure your wrists are under your shoulders and your knees are under your hips. Spread your fingers wide. Tuck your toes under and straighten your legs and arms, bringing your body into a straight line from the top of your head through the bottoms of your heels. Keep your stomach nice and strong and lift the front of your thighs up. Stay here for ten long, deep breaths. If this is too intense feel free to gently lower your knees to the floor. Always make sure you can breathe easily during this pose.

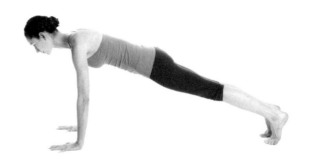

Plank Push-Up

You can do this with your knees either lifted or lowered, for a slightly less challenging version. Listen to your body. Bend your elbows straight back and lower your body halfway down in one straight line until your upper arms are parallel to the ground. If a half push-up is too intense you can either lower your knees so they're touching the ground and then bend your elbows to lower halfway, or slowly lower all the way down to your belly by simply bending your elbows straight back. Press straight up to plank.

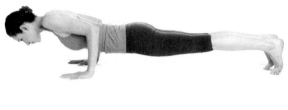

Side Plank with Tree

From your plank, lift your hips, press down with your right hand, roll to the outside edge of your right foot, and open your body to the left. Bend your left knee and place the bottom of your foot on your right upper thigh. Open your left arm straight up over your shoulders and look up at your hand. Stay here for five long, deep breaths, then repeat on the other side.

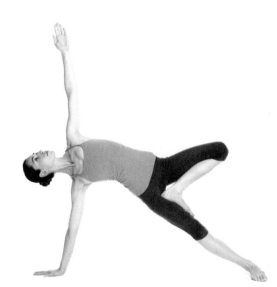

Crow

Come into a full squat. Press your palms firmly into the ground a few inches in front of your feet. Place your knees onto the tops of your upper arms. Look out about a foot ahead of you. Lift your hips and belly up. Stay here for a few breaths. If you feel steady lift one foot off the ground and place it back down. Then try lifting the other foot and placing it back down. If you are still stable, try lifting one foot, and then the other. Press down through your palms to lift both feet up, if possible. Stay here for three long, deep breaths and slowly lower your feet back down.

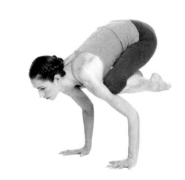

Scattered Mind

A scattered mind is all over the place and hard to rein in, even when called upon. Have you ever felt that you were working on several things at once but not really getting anything done fully? If you find yourself writing an e-mail while simultaneously checking Facebook and Twitter, snacking, and planning the next day's agenda, you're surely not being as efficient as you could be if you focused on one thing at a time. Being in a million places at once but not really focused on one is a scattered mind. You can self-diagnose it on the yoga mat. If you are in down dog and focused on the next pose, and then thinking about dinner, and your presentation, and back to being concerned about the next pose, you probably have a scattered mind.

At a conference of the American College of Sports Medicine, two researchers presented a paper showing that yoga can reduce anxiety, improve concentration, and increase motivation in as little as eight weeks. Traci A. Statler and Amy Wheeler tested students taking ten-week yoga classes at California State University, San Bernardino. The results were dramatic. "We were surprised by the degree of difference in just eight weeks of practice," said Statler. "We measured significant increases in all three areas."

THE SCATTERED MIND YOGA CURE

The cure for a scattered mind is to give it something to focus on for an extended period of time, and practice cooling yoga poses that calm down your nervous system. Do this routine daily.

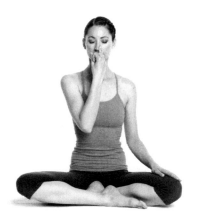

Alternate Nostril Breathing

Sit up tall, however you can sit comfortably. Take your right hand and curl down your index and middle finger into your palm. For this exercise you'll use your ring finger and your thumb.

Press your ring finger over your left nostril and inhale for four counts through your right nostril. Close off your right nostril with your thumb so both nostrils are closed. Hold all the air in for four counts. Release your ring finger and let all the air out your left nostril for four counts. Reverse this pattern starting with inhaling through the left nostril, holding both closed, and exhaling out the right side. Repeat this breathing pattern for three to five minutes.

Pigeon (torso release)

Come into a low lunge with your right leg forward. Scoot your right foot over toward your left hand and ease your right knee to the ground by your right hand. Rest your hips on the ground or on a blanket or pillow. Your hips and shoulders should be working themselves toward facing forward. Stay here for ten long, deep breaths. Gently lower your torso forward over your legs. If it feels good, make a pillow with your hands and rest your forehead on the tops of your hands. Stay here for ten long, deep breaths.

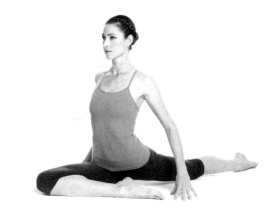

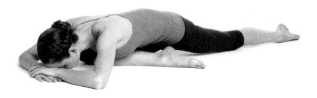

Shin Splints

Common in runners and other athletes, shin splints—causing shooting, burning pain in your shins—are a painful but frequent outcome of overuse. The discomfort in the front of the leg can be felt during exercise, or even constantly in some cases. Whichever you experience, shin splints can put a damper on your training regimen. Rest and icing are usually prescribed for shin splints, but some very gentle yoga poses can also help ease the pain.

THE SHIN SPLINTS YOGA CURE

The yoga cure for shin splints is a series of very mild, gentle movements that are designed to relieve pressure in the shins.

Hero

Stand on your knees so they are aligned under your hips. Press the tops of your feet down and into the ground. Press your thumbs into your legs, behind your knees, open your calves out to the sides and sit your hips down to the ground. Reach your knees forward. Stay here for ten long, deep breaths.

Hero, Reclined

If you feel like you have more room to work within this pose, slowly lower your back to the ground and reach your arms overhead. Continue to press down through the tops of your feet and reach forward through your knees. Stay here for ten long, deep breaths and slowly bring yourself up and out of the pose.

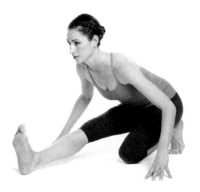

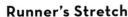

Runner's Stretch

Come into a low lunge with your right foot forward. Tuck the toes of your back foot under and lower your back knee to the ground. Shift your hips back to sit on your back heel. Your right leg should be straight in front of you. Relax your torso over your front leg. Stay here for five long, deep breaths. Bring yourself back to your lunge and do the same thing with the other leg.

Sugar Cravings

Cravings are another manifestation of tension and stress. A wandering, racing mind is susceptible to all kinds of misaligned thinking. A craving for sugar may stem from your body and mind feeling sluggish and wanting a boost of energy. If you eat a lot of sugar regularly, the cravings only intensify. Now, there's nothing terrible about having a little sugar every once in a while. Depriving ourselves of food and beating ourselves up over cravings can lead to all kinds of other issues, even disorders. Try making a healthy choice the next time a sugar craving hits, like having some hot tea with raw honey or a piece of dark chocolate, which can help lower blood pressure and maintain overall heart health.

When the cravings are out of control, and becoming an unhealthy regular occurrence, try this routine. Like all yoga, it's designed to tune you in to what's going on inside you.

THE SUGAR CRAVING YOGA CURE

Cravings and addictions have to do with not being in the present moment, and often not wanting to be. This is where the vice comes in, whether it is sugar, other foods, drugs, or alcohol. Yoga is all about being in the present moment and paying attention to what is going on with you, right now. Dealing with it is more useful in healing addictions and facing cravings than mindlessly masking our feelings with food, drugs, or alcohol.

This routine is designed to bring your attention away from cravings and back in touch with your breath, and in tune with your body. Do this routine three times a week to cure the cravings.

Seated Meditation Arms in V

Starting in a comfortable seated position, raise your arms overhead into in a V shape. Relax your shoulders down your back and reach out through your fingertips. We are going to stay and breathe here for three minutes. Finding the ease in staying here for several minutes will clear your mind and release loads of tension from your body.

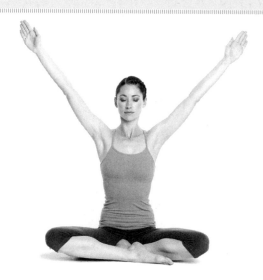

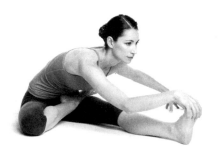

Seated One Leg Forward Bend (foot on hip crease)

Sit up tall with your shoulders above your hips. Extend your left leg straight out in front of you. Bend your right knee and place the top of your right foot on your left hip crease. If this hurts your knee or hip at all place your foot on the ground inside your left thigh instead. If your foot is on your hip crease, you should feel your heel pressing into your lower belly. Inhale and lift your arms straight up. As you exhale, fold your torso forward over your legs, keeping your spine long. Stay here for ten long, deep breaths.

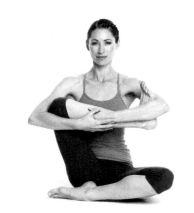

Seated Shin Hug

Hug your right knee with your arms. If there is room press the bottom of your right foot into your left elbow, wrap your right arm around your right thigh, and join your hands to cradle the leg. If that hurts your knee, hold your right foot with your left hand and your right knee with your right hand. Lengthen your torso and sit up tall. Relax your shoulders downward. Sway your left leg from side to side to open your hip.

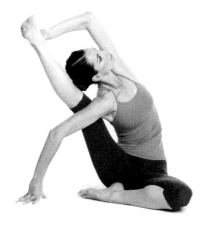

Compass

If your hips feel open, press your right hand under your right calf and bring your right leg to rest on top of your right shoulder. Grab the outside of your right foot with your left hand. Press your right fingertips into the ground alongside your right hip. Lean right, look under your left arm, and gaze upward. If there is room in your hamstrings, begin to straighten your right leg and keep opening your torso upward and toward your left. If it stops at the right upper arm, that's fine. Stay here for five long deep breaths. Unwind out of it and do the routine on the other side, beginning with the forward bend.

Tension

Tension likes to build up in our bodies and minds all day long. It's a natural part of life. Centuries ago, humans had stressful living conditions. How would you like to spend the day running for your life from predators and struggling for daily survival? Although our modern tensions may appear a bit different, we endure tension and stress in our bodies just the same as our ancestors did. The more stressful our day, the more tension builds. If we don't let the tension loose it will start to take a toll on us. It's important to tame tension each day so we can avoid heavy buildups that lead to sickness.

THE TENSION YOGA CURE

Managing tension doesn't necessarily mean finding ways to extinguish it. There will always be tension. How we deal with it, and how we manage it, is what matters in our lives. When we can find the ease within the effort and stress, we are able to manage a whole lot more with a lot less effort. Do this routine once or twice a day to press the reboot button and bring yourself back to a clean and neutral state.

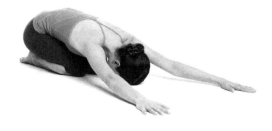

Child's Pose

Gently come onto all fours. Relax your hips and sit back on your heels. Rest your forehead on the ground and breathe deeply into your back. Stay here for five long, deep breaths.

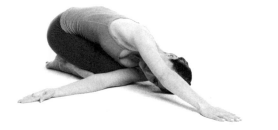

Child's Pose Twist

From your child's pose, thread your left arm under your right arm so your whole left shoulder is resting on the ground and the left side of your face is resting on the ground. Stay here for five long, deep breaths and do the same on the other side.

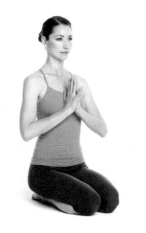

Sit on Heels, Palm Press
(lifting and lowering breath)

From your child's pose, sit up on your heels. Press your palms together in front of your chest, thumbs pressing into your sternum so you can feel your heart pumping. Close your eyes. See if you can slow down your heartbeat by deepening your breath. Take a big inhale, lifting your chest. Exhale all the air out through your mouth. Repeat this same breath and movement pattern twice more. Stay here and breathe naturally for a few more moments. When you're ready, gently relax your hands on your thighs.

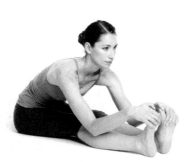

Seated, Both Legs Straight Forward

Sit up tall and bring both legs straight out in front of you. Inhale and lift your arms up. As you exhale, lengthen your torso forward and fold over your legs. If you can't hold your toes easily, bend your knees so your belly can rest on your thighs. You'll get a better opening with bent knees than by rounding your back and forcing your hands to your feet. Stay here for ten long, deep breaths.

Thyroid Imbalance

A regular yoga practice regulates all the systems of the body, and also corrects imbalances before they can become serious problems. B.K.S. Iyengar was one of the first modern yogis to describe the significance of shoulder stands in regulating the body's health; he recommends practicing them daily. Iyengar says the shoulder stand is a panacea for most common ailments, since it increases blood supply to the thyroid and parathyroid glands due to the chin lock in the neck region. Also the inverted position of the legs over the heart promotes healthy blood flow to help your body function efficiently.

THE THYROID IMBALANCE YOGA CURE

It's important to identify exactly what kind of thyroid imbalance you are dealing with, as each requires different support. Hyperthyroidism is a condition in which your thyroid gland produces too much of the hormone thyroxine, which can significantly accelerate your body's metabolism, causing sudden weight loss, a rapid or irregular heartbeat, sweating, and nervousness. Hypothyroidism is a condition characterized by abnormally low thyroid hormone production. Symptoms include sensitivity to cold, depression, fatigue, joint or muscle pain, dry skin, and unintentional weight gain.

Your thyroid hormone affects growth, development, and many cellular processes of the body, so having a healthy thyroid has a lot more to do with the overall health of your body than how slowly or quickly your body is able to metabolize food. This routine is designed to regulate your thyroid gland and bring you back into a balanced state.

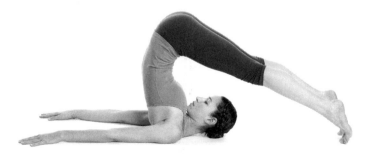

Plow

Lie down on your back with your arms at your sides. Press down into your arms, round your back, and slowly bring your feet over your head. If this puts too much tension on your back or neck, roll out of it slowly and relax. Don't force your neck in this position. If your back and neck feel okay, stay here for ten long, deep breaths.

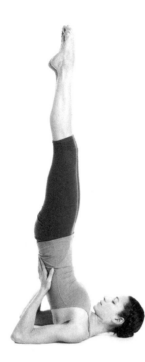

Shoulder Stand

If your neck feels pretty tight in your plow, stay there a little longer and then slowly roll back down to lie on your back. If your neck feels good in plow, press your palms into your back so your fingers face up. Wiggle your elbows closer together and scoot your hands up your back, close to your shoulders. Lift the backs of your legs straight up so your body is in one straight line. Stay here for twenty long, deep breaths. Either close your eyes or keep your gaze softly resting on your belly button.

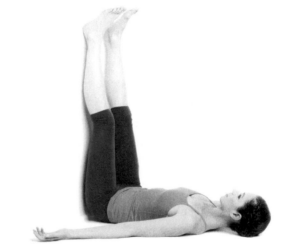

Legs Up the Wall

Sit facing a wall. Bring your hips right up to the wall. Lie down so your torso is perpendicular to the wall. Bring your legs up the wall. Stay here for five minutes.

Reclining Butterfly

Lie down on your back. Bring the bottoms of your feet together and let your knees relax out to the sides. Rest your hands either down by your sides or on top of your thighs, whichever is most comfortable for you. Stay here for twenty long, deep breaths.

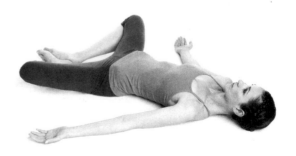

Traveler's Anxiety

Air travel can serve up a load of anxiety. Whether you get anxious about traveling, flying, the stress of airports, lines, crowds, or just being stuck in an airplane for hours, there are plenty of opportunities between getting to and from your destination for stress to creep in.

Fear of flying is essentially an anxiety disorder. We can control our fears by bringing our attention back to the breath.

Even if you have little or no fear of flying, being in an airplane, especially if you are a regular traveler, can take a toll on your health. The cabin pressure, being cooped up in a seat for hours, and the recycled oxygen aren't ideal conditions for our bodies or minds. Luckily, there are some simple yoga poses and techniques you can do right from your seat on the airplane that will release tension in your body and settle your mind.

THE TRAVELER'S ANXIETY YOGA CURE: AIRPLANE YOGA

You can do this routine from your seat in the airplane. It will reduce anxiety and open up the spine. Also, try to get up and walk around. On long flights, try to get up every hour for a walk. Don't be shy about striking a tree pose when you're waiting in line for the bathroom. Who knows, your fellow passengers just may join in!

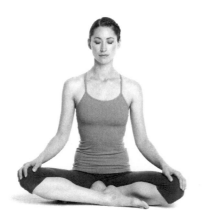

Seated Meditation

Sit up tall in your chair with both feet flat on the floor, with your knees facing forward and over your toes. Relax your shoulders, so that they are away from your ears. Rest your hand on your thighs and close your eyes. Start to rest your attention on your breath. Watch your inhales come and exhales go. Settle your mind in the space between. Begin to lengthen and deepen your inhales and exhales, making them longer and setting an easy pace of breathing. If a thought starts to enter your mind, simply observe it like a cloud passing by. Continue observing your breath for three to five minutes.

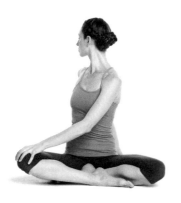

Seated Easy Twist

From your comfortable, seated position, inhale and lift your left arm up. As you exhale, rest your left hand on your right knee. Press your right fingertips into the seat behind your hips. Inhale and lengthen your torso up tall. Exhale and twist your torso around to the right. At the bottom of your exhale return your torso to center and repeat the same movement and breathing pattern on the other side.

THE TRAVELER'S ANXIETY YOGA CURE: HOTEL YOGA

When you arrive at your destination, try to make some time to do yoga in your hotel room, or wherever you are staying. Even five minutes of simple sun salutations will help to reenergize the body and get your circulation going again. Yoga is a fantastic cure for jet lag, too!

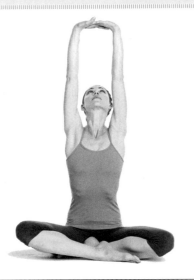

Seated Palm Press

Staying seated, interlace your hands and press your palms straight up overhead. Relax your shoulders down your back and look up toward your fingers. Stay here for three long, deep breaths, and gently relax your hands down by your sides.

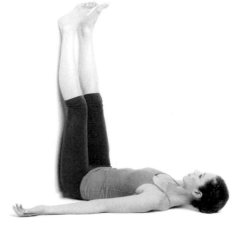

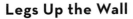

Legs Up the Wall

After you've finished your sun salutations, relaxing with your legs up the wall will regulate blood flow and reduce pressure in your body while simultaneously calming your mind. Sit facing a wall. Bring your hips right up to the wall. Lie down so your torso is perpendicular to the wall. Bring your legs up the wall. Stay here for five minutes.

Tummy Trouble

Tummy trouble is uncomfortable, sometimes painful, and absolutely no fun. Whether your digestion is having a hard time getting a move on, or your stomach is in a knot from stress, or something else is going on in there, these simple yoga poses can soothe a troubled tummy in a flash and get you back to feeling great again. If tummy trouble persists, you could have a more serious condition than a bellyache, so make sure to see your doctor.

THE TUMMY TROUBLE YOGA CURE

The yoga cure for tummy trouble is to take it easy. Especially if your tummy is irritated and your insides are screaming at you, this routine is designed to calm down your system from the inside out. You will be left with a calm and happy tummy so you can go about your life pain free.

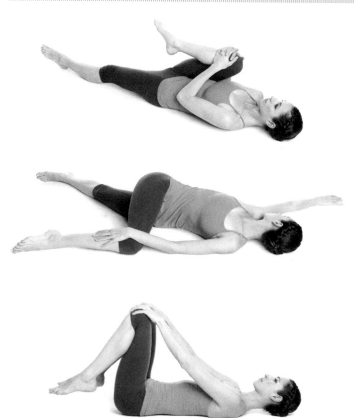

Reclining Single Knee Hug

Lie down on your back. Hug your right knee gently into your chest. With each exhale, draw your knee closer toward your right shoulder. Stay here for five long, deep breaths.

Reclining Single Knee Hug Twist

From your reclining knee hug, cross your right knee over your body toward your left. Open your arms out to the sides. Look toward your right. Stay here for ten long, deep breaths. Do the other side starting with the reclining knee hug.

Rock

Draw both knees into your chest. Gently rock from side to side allowing the sides of your back to release into the ground. Continue rocking for five long, deep breaths.

Under-Eye Bags and Dark Circles

A common cause of under-eye bags and dark circles is not getting enough rest or proper nutrition. Salty and processed foods may cause you to retain water and make puffy eyes worse. Some experts say that under-eye bags are a natural part of the aging process, caused by weakened ligaments making the natural fat under the eyes push forward and form a puffy bag. It's a good thing we know that yoga can reverse the effects of aging.

As I've said repeatedly, a regular yoga practice makes you gravitate naturally toward healthier food choices and also helps you sleep a lot better, so you should be on your way to eliminating puffy eyes and dark circles as soon as you step onto your mat. The key is to keep doing it every day. It only works if you practice.

THE UNDER-EYE BAGS AND DARK CIRCLES YOGA CURE

The yoga cure for under-eye bags and dark circles is to first take a look at how you are living your life. If you can get more sleep, eat healthier, drink more water, and think happier, less stressed thoughts, begin there. Inversions literally bring more blood to your head and improve the health and appearance of your facial skin. Any time your head is below your heart in yoga you are improving blood flow and refreshing the skin of the face. Inversions and some other calming poses included here will yield you the most benefits.

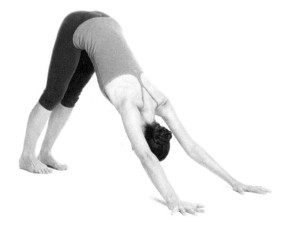

Down Dog

From all fours, tuck your toes, lift your hips, and press back into down dog. Reach your heels toward the ground. Relax your shoulders toward the ground and relax your head and neck. Stay here for five long, deep breaths.

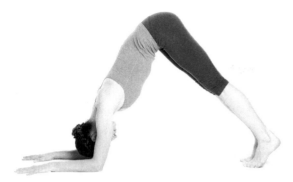

Forearm Down Dog

From your down dog, lower your forearms to the ground so they are parallel to each other. Keep your fingers spread wide. Lift your shoulders away from the ground and relax your head. Stay here for five long, deep breaths.

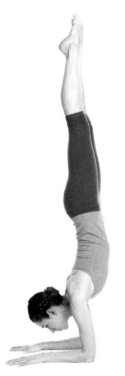

Forearm Stand

If you would like to move into a forearm stand, inhale and lift your right leg up so that your hips lift over your shoulders. Exhale and lower it back down. Try the same thing with the left leg. Continue with this until you get the feeling of getting your hips over your shoulders, or if you feel ready, take a light hop the next time you inhale and lift a leg to bring yourself into forearm stand. If you are new to the pose, try positioning yourself near a wall so you can kick up and rest your legs along the wall. Stay here for five long, deep breaths and slowly lower down to child's pose.

Calm Eyes

Sit up nice and tall, however you can sit comfortably. Rub the palms of your hands together pretty quickly to get a good amount of heat going. Close your eyes and gently press the heels of your hands into your eyelids. Rest your fingers against your forehead. Stay here for three long, deep breaths and gently relax your hands to rest on your thighs.

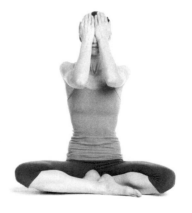

Vertigo

The feeling of dizziness and spinning when you are stationary that comes with vertigo is no fun. The lost balance that comes when vertigo strikes can be both scary and dangerous. It can be caused by an inner ear imbalance, anxiety, and even problems in the brain, so it's important to see your doctor if you are experiencing vertigo. In many cases, yoga can help ease the anxiety that comes with this condition; it also has been known to balance out the body's systems to reduce and even cure it.

THE VERTIGO YOGA CURE

The yoga cure for vertigo is to breathe really deeply and move super slowly, knowing that you always have the option to stop and back out of a pose. Sitting up on your heels or resting in child's pose are great places to be if you have a dizzy spell. If you feel light-headed or the room starts spinning, always back out of a pose.

Plow

Lie down on your back with your arms at your sides. Press down into your arms, round your back, and slowly bring your feet over your head. If this puts too much tension on your back or neck, roll out of it slowly and relax. Don't force your neck in this position. If your back and neck feel okay, stay here for ten long, deep breaths.

Shoulder Stand

Slowly roll back down to lie on your back. Press your palms into your back so your fingers face up. Wiggle your elbows closer together and scoot your hands up your back close to your shoulders. Lift the backs of your legs straight up so your body is in one straight line. Stay here for twenty long, deep breaths. Either close your eyes or keep your gaze softly resting on your belly button.

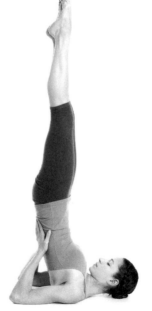

Headstand Prep

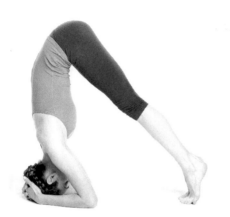

Sit on your heels with your shoulders above your hips. Interlace your fingers loosely and place them on the ground. Place the top of your head on the ground so your fingers hold the back of your head. Stay here for a few breaths to get comfortable in the position. If you can, stay here for a few breaths before you back out. If you are comfortable, tuck your toes and straighten your legs like you would in a down dog. Stay here for ten long, deep breaths and when you are ready to come out of it, gently lower your knees to the ground and relax in child's pose.

Child's Pose

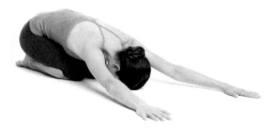

Gently come onto all fours. Relax your hips and sit back on your heels. Rest your forehead on the ground and breathe deeply into your back. Stay here for five long, deep breaths.

Sit on Heels

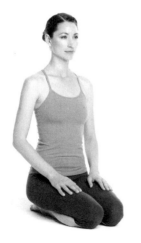

From your child's pose, keeping your hips on your heels, sit up so your shoulders are aligned above your hips. Rest your palms on your thighs. Stay here for five long, deep breaths.

Wrinkles

If we're lucky, we will live long enough for time to eventually wrinkle our skin. These wrinkles tell the story of our lives. It's up to us if our faces are going to tell a tale of years spent smiling and laughing, or days wasted frowning and scowling. How we view and deal with aging is up to us. A healthy and joyful relationship with ourselves as time goes by is much more useful and lovely than spending our adult years chasing after a vanished youth. There is no point. Chasing after a ghost of ourselves only leads to more misaligned thought patterns, habits, and actions . . . and to unhappiness in our own skin, literally.

Enjoy today! We only get to live each day once. Enjoy each moment fully. Aging is a natural and beautiful part of life. Wrinkles don't have to be the kiss of death or something we rush to smooth out with aggressive skin treatments or plastic surgery. Enjoy who you are today and every day.

That being said, taking great care of your skin will keep you vibrant and fresh from the inside out. You can't buy a skin cream that provides the glow you get from happy, healthy insides. Only you can light up your skin from the inside. Yoga can show you how. Yoga can keep your skin glowing, reduce the effects of gravity, and keep the stresses in your life from making you haggard.

Tonya Jacobs, a scientist at UC Davis's Center for Mind and Brain, reported that meditators show improved psychological well-being, and that these improvements lead to biochemical changes associated with resistance to aging at the cellular level. You can change your body at the cellular level with yoga. Also, the more yoga you practice, the less you'll make scrunched-up faces from being in an unpleasant mood. Repetitive frown and stress lines, gone!

THE WRINKLES YOGA CURE

The yoga cure for wrinkles is to not care when you get wrinkles. You've earned them through living. The cure for getting wrinkles that you don't need is being happy, less stressed, and practicing yoga regularly.

This routine is designed to relax you as well as reverse the effects of gravity on your body. Stay easy and calm when you practice. If you have a hard time staying calm, stop wherever you are and take a long, deep inhale through the nose, and exhale through the mouth. Repeat twice more for a nice, settling effect.

Practice this routine daily to revitalize yourself from the inside out.

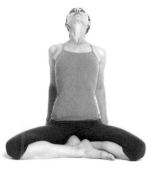

Seated Chest Lift

From a comfortable, seated position, press your fingertips into the ground behind your hips. Inhale and lift your chest up. If it feels good, lengthen your hips up off the ground also, creating lots of space between each of your vertebrae. As you exhale, gently lower your hips back down and sit up tall.

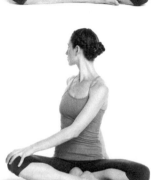

Seated Easy Twist

From your comfortable, seated position, inhale and lift your left arm up. As you exhale, rest your left hand on your right knee. Press your right fingertips into the ground behind your hips. Inhale and lengthen your torso up tall. Exhale and twist your torso around to the right. At the bottom of your exhale return your torso to center and repeat the same movement and breathing pattern on the other side.

Headstand

If you are new to the headstand pose it's best to attempt with the assistance of a yoga teacher or someone who has been doing yoga for a while and can help.

Sit on your heels with your shoulders above your hips. Interlace your fingers loosely and place them on the ground. Place the top of your head on the ground so your fingers hold the back of your head. Stay here for a few breaths to get comfortable in the position. Tuck your toes and straighten your legs like you would in a down dog. Stay here for ten long, deep breaths and when you are ready to come out of it, gently lower your knees to the ground and relax in child's pose.

Start to walk your feet in toward your body so your hips line up over your shoulders and your back is vertical. Stay here for a few breaths. If you are comfortable here bend one knee in and bring your heel to your hip. Bring it back down and try the other leg. Try both legs at the same time. When your heels are pulled in toward your hips, slowly extend your legs straight up. Stay for twenty long, deep breaths if you can. When you are ready to come down slowly lower one leg at a time and rest in child's pose for a few breaths.

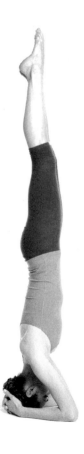

Zzzs (Getting Some)

Getting to sleep and staying asleep have developed into major problems that interrupt the daily lives of millions. Prescriptions for sleeping medications topped 56 million in 2008, up 54 percent from 2004. A regular yoga practice can completely cure the condition for many, turning an insomniac into someone who sleeps like a baby and wakes up refreshed and energized. In 2004, Harvard researcher Sat Bir Singh Khalsa, published a study that found that a half hour to forty-five minutes of daily yoga helped chronic insomniacs get to sleep and stay asleep throughout the night. For twenty participants, sleep was significantly improved. Yoga works. Yoga cures.

Our minds inform the functions of our bodies. With yoga we learn we can control and relax the mind to move through various poses with ease. We can also ease the mind to sleep well at night. When we practice yoga regularly, many of the anxieties and triggers that keep us up at night simply melt away, and we can sink into our sheets with ease.

THE ZZZS (GETTING SOME) YOGA CURE

The yoga cure for insomnia is simple: begin and maintain a regular yoga practice.

In addition to a regular yoga practice, a little yoga right before bed will help to wind you down so you can sleep great right through the night. This routine is designed to calm the mind and release any lasting tension in the body at bedtime.

You can do it on the ground beside your bed or even right in bed if you prefer.

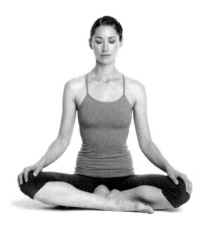

Seated Meditation

Sit up nice and tall, however you can sit most comfortably. If you have a headboard on your bed, lean against it. Relax your shoulders, so that they are away from your ears. Rest your hands on your thighs and close your eyes. Start to rest your attention on your breath. Watch your inhales come and exhales go. Settle your mind in the space between. Begin to lengthen and deepen your inhales and exhales, setting a slow, easy pace of breathing. If a thought starts to enter your mind, simply observe it like a cloud passing by. Continue observing your breath for three to five minutes.

Reclined Single Knee Hug Twist

Gently, lie down on your back. Hug your right knee into your chest. Twist your right leg over toward your left side. Relax your arms out to the sides. Stay here for ten long, deep breaths and repeat on the other side.

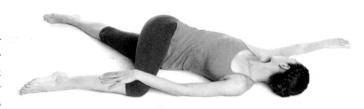

Reclined Hamstring Release

Return to lying down. Gently hug your right knee into your chest. Extend your right leg straight up and hold the back of your hamstring or knee. Allow your leg to relax closer to your face with each exhale. Try to avoid pulling the leg with your arms. Just allow your breath to release the tension and move it closer to you naturally. Stay here for ten long, deep breaths. Repeat on the other side.

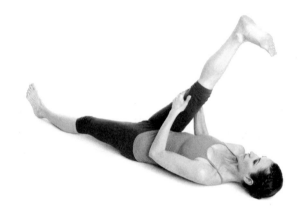

Happy Baby

Return to lying down. Hug both knees into your chest. Grab the outside edge of your right foot with your right hand and do the same with your left foot and hand. Point the bottoms of your feet straight up to the ceiling. Gently pull your knees down toward the ground by pulling your feet down. Rock your body from side to side to release tension in your hips and back. Stay here for five long, deep breaths and return to lying down.

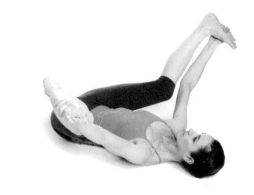

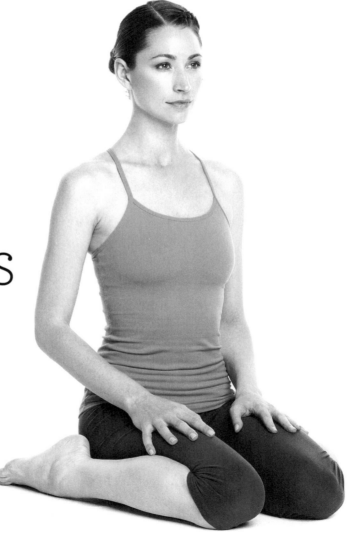

Bonus Material:

Designing Your Own AT-HOME YOGA RETREATS

By now you know that the more you can integrate yoga into your daily life, the happier and healthier you will be. One thing that can help you do this in a meaningful and lasting way is to create an inspirational environment in your home, one that reminds you to take a deep breath and connect back to yourself. Yoga can then be carried with you throughout your day—whether you're lounging, relaxing, working, or anything in between.

I like to joke at Strala that practicing yoga is like moving into a bigger house or apartment inside yourself, without the increase in rent or mortgage. You feel better after a yoga practice because your body has more room and your head is a little clearer.

Home is a great place to practice yoga. With a few simple ideas and yoga routines, you can transform your home into a year-round yoga retreat, allowing you to renew and inspire yourself and your creativity every day.

Want to cleanse your entire system and declutter your home while you're at it, giving yourself a fresh start from the inside out? Then the two-day detox and declutter retreat is on the menu. Are you looking for a bit of inspiration to make a creative shift in your life? I have just the inspiration retreat set up for you. Would you rather kick back, relax, and rejuvenate? If so, the relax, restore, and rejuvenate retreat is suited especially to you. Pick your retreat or do all three. All you need is a weekend and you're on your way to sheer bliss. Get it on the calendar! Happy retreating!

Detox and Declutter Retreat

Your home is your place of peaceful, calm, grounded energy in which you should feel safe and relaxed. If your home is cluttered and messy it's nearly impossible to feel at peace. There are a few simple adjustments that you can make to create calm in your home that don't require pricey remodeling, installation of life-size Buddha statues, or digging a koi pond equipped with a tranquil waterfall.

CLEAN AND DETOX

Most of us have clutter to one degree or another in our homes. I confess that I have been known to let papers and books pile up with the excuse that I need them sprawled out so I can look at them for reference and inspiration. The truth is, they get piled up so high and are often scattered so widely that at times I wouldn't be able to find an important letter, book, or unpaid bill if I didn't engage in emergency decluttering. So let's just say that I personally understand the benefits of decluttering from the inside out and the outside in. Body/mind/home: there are more connections than we might like to admit!

Confronting clutter can be daunting. Where to begin? When we open our eyes and actually pay attention to what is around us in our homes we can start to look at what we need, what we don't, and what we need to organize. We all have the ability to create calm in our homes and lives. We can treat cleaning and decluttering the home like a yoga practice that cleans and declutters the mind. Both practices require daily attention and repetition.

When you practice clearing the clutter you are making room for inspiration and creativity to rush in and fill the space (without taking up more room). We need to make space inside and out. So let's get started doing it.

DAY 1: WRITE IT DOWN

Start your retreat in the morning. You'll need a notebook and a pen. Sit up tall, where you can sit comfortably, your favorite spot in your home. Take a long, deep inhale and exhale. Look around your house. Is there a lot of clutter around that you can easily put away? Are there piles of mail, laundry, and stuff? Write down where you see the clutter and make a plan for what you are going to do with it. Do you need to go through the piles, do the laundry, or stack old clothes to go to a donation center? Make a list and make a plan.

Now, close your eyes and begin to rest your attention on your breath. If your mind starts to wander toward thinking, gently guide it back. Ask yourself the following questions:

- How is my health?
- What can I do to improve my health?
- Do I eat things that are not healthy?
- Could I eat more healthfully?
- How is my anxiety level?
- Could I be less stressed?
- What could I do daily to reduce my stress levels?

Open your eyes and write down whatever comes to mind in your notebook. Finding out what might be cluttering up your health is important, so write freely here. Take a look at what you have written. Come up with a plan for clearing the clutter in your house that's getting in the way of living healthfully. If you have time, begin clearing now. Even if you only have a chance to take care of one stack of papers, take care of that one stack.

Yoga to Declutter: Morning Routine

Do this routine after you've done your writing and your decluttering.

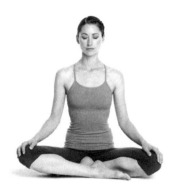

Seated Meditation

Sit up nice and tall, however you can sit most comfortably. Relax your shoulders, so that they are away from your ears. Rest your hands on your thighs and close your eyes. Start to rest your attention on your breath. Watch your inhales come and exhales go. Settle your mind in the space between. Begin to lengthen and deepen your inhales and exhales setting a slow, easy pace of breathing. If a thought starts to enter your mind, simply observe it like a cloud passing by. Continue observing your breath for three to five minutes.

Breath of Fire

Staying seated, take a long and deep inhale. Exhale all of the air out. Begin to breathe rapidly in and out through the nose. Pick up the pace if you can and keep your inhales and exhales even. Continue for one minute. After a minute slow down your inhales and exhales gradually until you come back to long and deep breathing. Gently open your eyes.

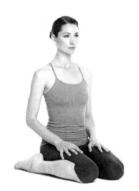

Hero

Stand on your knees and lift your hips up over your knees. Bring your thumbs to the backs of your knees and move your calves out to the sides. Press down into the ground firmly with the tops of your feet. Sit your hips down on the ground between your feet. If your hips don't reach the ground easily or this hurts your knees at all, sit on a pillow or a block. Continue to press the tops of your feet down toward the ground to protect the knees. Stay here for ten long, deep breaths.

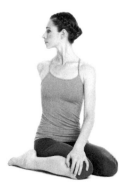

Hero Twist

Staying in your hero pose, bring your left hand to hold your right knee. Press your right fingertips into the ground behind your hips. Inhale and lengthen your torso up tall. Exhale and twist your torso further to the right.

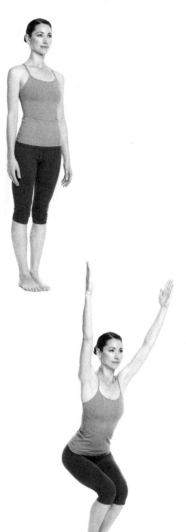

Standing

Stand at the top of your yoga mat. Feet are parallel and slightly apart, under your hip bones. Your hip bones aren't at the outside of your hips so make sure your feet aren't too far apart. You can check by placing two fists between your feet. That's about the width of your hip bones. Close your eyes and bring your attention to your breath. Lengthen and deepen your inhales and exhales and continue breathing at this nice long pace for five full breaths. Gently open your eyes.

Chair with Breath of Fire

Inhale and sink your hips low as you reach your arms above your shoulders. Relax your shoulders down your back and lengthen through your sides. Stay here for three long, deep breaths. Add breath of fire for thirty seconds.

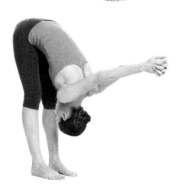

Standing Forward Bend Shoulder Opener

From your chair pose, fold your torso over your legs, interlace your hands behind your back, and relax your shoulders. Let your arms fall toward the ground with each exhale. If your hamstrings feel tense, bend your knees and rest your belly on your thighs. Stay here for five long, deep breaths.

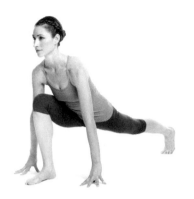

Low Lunge

Press both fingertips into the ground, bend your knees, and step your left leg back to a low lunge. Sink your hips low. Lengthen out forward through the top of your head and back through your left heel. If it feels good to you, move your body a little, side to side and front to back, to allow your hips to open up and soften. Stay here for five long, deep breaths.

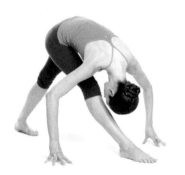

Single Leg Forward Bend

From the last pose, press your fingertips into the floor by either side of your legs. Step your left leg back a couple feet behind your right leg. Straighten both legs and fold your torso over your front leg. If your front leg doesn't straighten easily, bend it enough so your fingers can press into the ground. Stay here for ten long, deep breaths and then repeat on the other side.

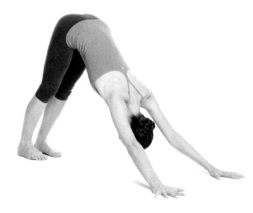

Down Dog

Bend your front leg slightly, press your palms firmly down on either side of your front foot, and step back to down dog. Relax your heels toward the ground. Relax your shoulders and head.

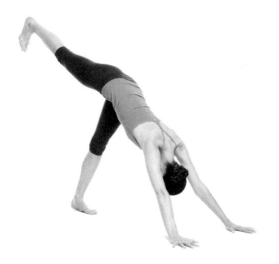

Down Dog Split

From your down dog, inhale as you lift your right leg high. Keep your hips square so your right toes point down toward the ground. Lift your right leg up from the back of your upper thigh. Press equally through both hands and heels. Keep your arms and legs straight.

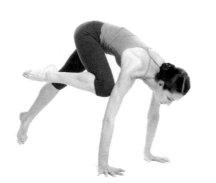

Down Dog Split, Knee to Shoulder

From your down dog split, keep your hips and stomach lifted high as you inhale and bring your right knee to touch your right shoulder. As you exhale, lift your leg back into the split.

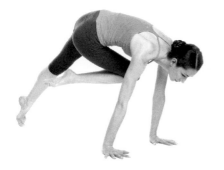

Down Dog Split, Knee Across

From your down dog split, keep your hips and stomach lifted high as you inhale and bring your right knee toward the back of your left upper arm. As you exhale, lift your leg back to your down dog split.

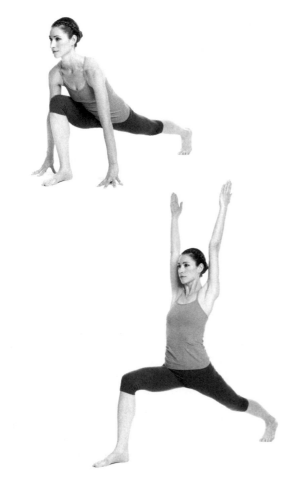

Low Lunge

From your down dog split, inhale and lift your right knee toward your forehead and place your foot between your hands. Sink your hips low. Lengthen out forward through the top of your head and back through your left heel. If it feels good to you, move your body a little, side to side and front to back, to allow your hips to open up and soften. Stay here for five long, deep breaths.

High Lunge Arms Up

Come into a low lunge. Press down through your feet and bring your torso up, aligning your shoulders above your hips. Inhale and lift your arms straight up. Relax your shoulders down your back. Stay here for five long, deep breaths.

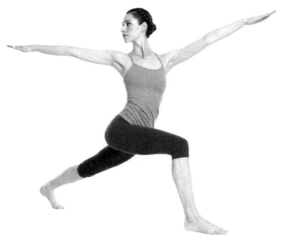

High Lunge Twist

From your high lunge, as you exhale, spin your body toward your right and open your arms out to the sides. Sink your hips low so your front thigh is parallel with the ground.

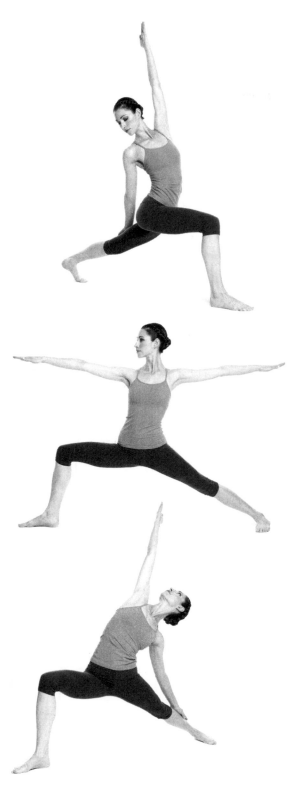

High Lunge Twist Reverse

From your high lunge twist, tip your torso back toward your back leg as you inhale. Let your right hand rest lightly on your back leg.

Warrior 2

From your high lunge twist reverse, spin your back heel down so the bottom of your foot is firmly planted on the ground. Windmill your arms overhead, open your torso to your left, bend your front knee over your front foot. Open your arms straight out and away from your torso, right arm in font of you, and left arm behind you, palms down. Look over your front hand. Bend your front knee over your front foot and sink your hips low so your right thigh is parallel to the ground. Stay here for ten long, deep breaths.

Reverse Warrior

From your warrior 2, inhale and lean your torso back, opening up your sides. Let your left hand graze and lightly rest on your back leg. Lengthen your right arm overhead. Stay here for two long, deep breaths.

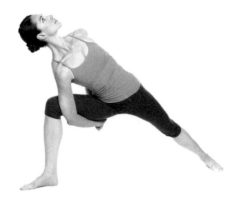

Extended Angle (bind)

From your reverse warrior, move your torso up and out over your front leg. Either press your right forearm onto your right thigh and lengthen your left arm overhead or if you can extend your torso to bind your arms around your leg (and doing so doesn't affect your long, deep breathing), wrap your arms around your right leg and open your torso up so your chest is lengthening up toward the ceiling. Stay here for five long, deep breaths.

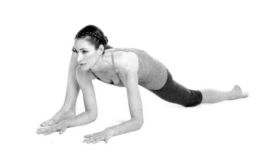

Lizard

From your last pose go into a low lunge, with your right leg forward. Move your right foot over toward your right hand, keeping your toes pointing forward. Lower your back knee down to the ground. Gently lower your forearms to the ground. Stay here for ten long, deep breaths.

From the lizard, press back to down dog, gently walk your feet up toward your hands, and roll up to standing. Repeat the routine up to here starting with standing. When you get to lizard on the other side, press back to down dog, gently walk your feet up toward your hands, bend your knees, and come to lie down on your back.

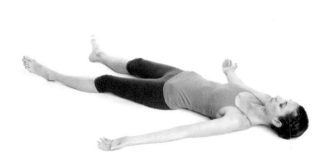

Corpse

Lie down on your back. Open your legs hip width apart, or a bit wider, depending on what's most comfortable for you. Relax your arms a bit out to your sides, palms facing up. Take a big inhale through your nose, and exhale all the air out through your mouth. Repeat this breathing pattern two more times. Then just lie there and relax for three to five minutes.

When you are ready to come out of it, slowly start to deepen your breath. Roll your wrists and ankles. Gently hug your knees into your chest and rock up to sitting.

BITES OF BLISS

Please attempt to eat very healthfully during your retreat...we want to remove the interior clutter, too. A few suggestions:

- **Water:** Drink a ton of water over the next two days. Water is nature's best cleanser, inside and out. Often we don't get enough. Keep a large glass refilled all day for the next two days. Keep a glass by your bed at night also.
- **Dandelion tea:** You can pick up the tea bags at most health food stores and a lot of major grocery stores. Drink the tea twice a day to help promote detoxification and cleanse the system.
- **Quinoa and kale:** A very tasty meal for lunch or dinner or both! Kale is a super food, very high in beta carotene, vitamins K and C, and lutein, and also rich in calcium. The antioxidants in kale have been linked to lower cholesterol and reduced risk for at least five types of cancer, including bladder, breast, colon, ovary, and prostate. Steam it to add to its cholesterol-lowering ability. Quinoa is as easy to cook as rice and is a complete protein, meaning it includes all nine essential amino acids. Quinoa is rich in lysine, which is essential for tissue growth and repair. Also high in magnesium, iron, copper, and phosphorus, quinoa is useful for combating headaches, symptoms of diabetes, and atherosclerosis.

After you finish your routine, go about your day as you normally would, and look for ways you can clear clutter from your life, physically and emotionally. If you would prefer to stay in "retreat mode," pick up an inspiring book you've been thinking about reading, read for a while, maybe take a nap, and go for a long walk. Enjoy a nice leisurely day without any tasks to concern yourself with.

Yoga to Declutter: Evening Routine

Do this routine at night either before or after you eat dinner. If you're doing it after dinner, give yourself at least an hour to digest your food.

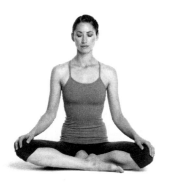

Seated Meditation

Sit up nice and tall, however you can sit most comfortably. Relax your shoulders, so that they are away from your ears. Rest your hands on your thighs and close your eyes. Start to rest your attention on your breath. Watch your inhales come and exhales go. Settle your mind in the space between. Begin to lengthen and deepen your inhales and exhales, setting a slow, easy pace of breathing. If a thought starts to enter your mind, simply observe it like a cloud passing by. Continue observing your breath for three to five minutes.

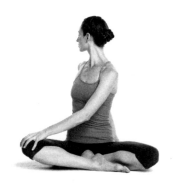

Seated Easy Twist

From your comfortable, seated position, inhale and lift your left arm up. As you exhale, rest your left hand on your right knee. Press your right fingertips into the ground behind your hips. Inhale and lengthen your torso up tall. Exhale and twist your torso around to the right. At the bottom of your exhale return your torso to center and repeat the same movement and breathing pattern on the other side.

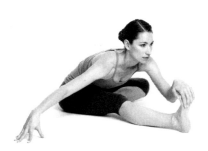

Seated One Leg Forward Bend

Sit up tall. Extend your right leg forward and flex your right foot. Bend your left foot in toward our body so your knee relaxes out toward the left side. Inhale and extend your arms straight up. Exhale and fold your torso over your right leg. Grab your right toes with your left hand and press your right fingertips on the ground beside your right leg. Lift your torso up and over your right leg. Extend the left side of your back out long. Stay here for ten long, deep breaths.

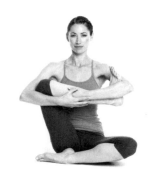

Seated Shin Hug

Hug your right knee with your arms so your shin is parallel to the ground. Bend your left knee and slide your leg in so your heel is close to the center of your body. Lengthen your torso and sit up tall. Relax your shoulders downward. Sway your shin and leg from side to side to open your hip.

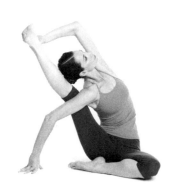

Compass

Press your right hand under your right calf and bring your right leg to rest on top of your right shoulder. Grab the outside of your right foot with your left hand. Press your right fingertips into the ground alongside your right hip. Lean right, look under your left arm, and gaze upward. Begin to straighten your right leg and keep opening your torso upward and toward your left. Stay here for five long, deep breaths. Unwind out of that and do the routine on the other side.

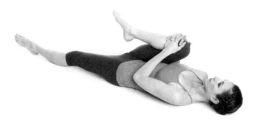

Reclining Single Knee Hug

Lie down on your back. Hug your right knee in toward your chest. With each exhale, draw your knee closer toward your right shoulder. Stay here for five long, deep breaths.

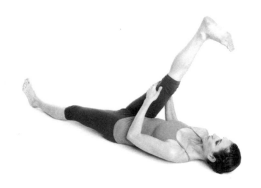

Reclining Hamstring Release

Extend your right leg upward. Grab behind your calf, your knee, or your hamstring, wherever you can grab easily. Stay here for ten long, deep breaths. Try not to pull the leg closer toward you, but instead allow your exhales to release tension and only move the leg closer when more space opens up.

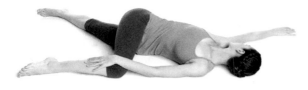

Reclining Single Knee Hug Twist

From your reclining knee hug, cross your right knee over your body toward your left. Open your arms out to the sides. Look toward your right. Stay here for ten long, deep breaths. Do the other side starting with the reclining knee hug.

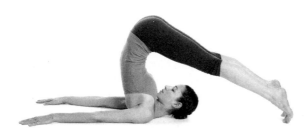

Plow

From lying down, press your arms down by your sides, round your back, and bring your feet over your head into a plow pose.

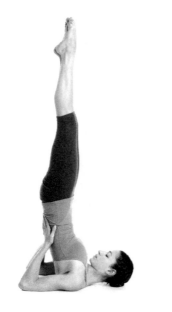

Shoulder Stand

Slowly roll back down to lie on your back. Press your palms into your back so your fingers face up. Wiggle your elbows closer together and scoot your hands up your back close to your shoulders. Lift the backs of your legs straight up so your body is in one straight line. Stay here for twenty long, deep breaths. Either close your eyes or keep your gaze softly resting on your belly button.

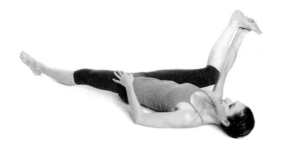

Half Happy Baby

Lie down on your back. Hug your right knee into your chest. Point the bottom of your foot straight up. Grab the outside edge of your right foot with your right hand. Press your right knee down toward the ground with the strength of your arm. Stay here for five long, deep breaths. Switch sides.

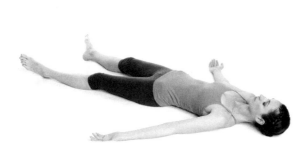

Corpse

Lie down on your back. Open your legs hip width, or a bit wider, depending on what's most comfortable for you. Relax your arms a bit out to your sides, palms facing up. Take a big inhale through your nose, exhale all the air out through your mouth. Repeat the same breathing pattern twice more. Relax your entire self for three to five minutes.

When you are ready to come out of it, slowly start to deepen your breath. Roll around your wrists and ankles. Gently hug your knees into your chest and rock up to sit up comfortably.

Try to keep distractions to a minimum before bedtime. Read a book or journal instead of watching TV or using the computer. Keep your journal by your bed in case you want to write down any thoughts. Sleep well!

DAY 2: WAKE AND REFLECT

When you first wake up, sit in bed and lean against the wall or your headboard if you have one. Relax your hands on your thighs and pay attention to your breath. Stay here and meditate for a few minutes. When you are finished, write down in your journal anything that comes to mind. If you have any thoughts about Day 1 of the retreat, write them down.

Before breakfast, do the morning routine. Go about your day as usual, doing what you need to get done; continue drinking lots of water and making healthy choices. If you have time, clear some more clutter in your home.

At night, before dinner, set aside ten minutes for meditation. Keep your journal handy. Write down any thoughts or inspirations that came up for you today. Sit up tall, comfortably, wherever you most like to sit in your home. Take a long and deep inhale and exhale. Close your eyes and simply follow your breath for ten minutes. Relax fully and watch your inhales come and your exhales go. If a thought or inspiration comes that you'd like to remember, write it down, and come back to your breath.

Perform the evening routine either before or after dinner. When it is bedtime, again try to avoid overstimulation like TV or staring at your computer screen. Read or write in your journal before bed. Keep your journal and a big glass of water by your bed.

When you wake up in the morning repeat the morning meditation and journal writing. This time after you've written down whatever first comes to mind, write about your experience over the last two days. If there is any part of the retreat you found useful that you can integrate into your daily life, write it down with the intention of doing so. Enjoy the rest of your day!

Inspiration Retreat

Inspiration sparks change and transformation. Whatever inspires you to make a shift in your life for the better, run with it and let it power you like jet fuel. Your inspiration will take you far. Feel a desire to refresh your life? Have a big life-changing event coming up? Whatever the circumstance, the next two days are designed to inspire you, and provide that spark we all need to keep us energized and excited by life.

We all go through phases of inspiration and lulls where it's a little harder to get up and get going. When going through a lull, there are simple things that you can do around your home to re-inspire yourself and invigorate your passions. When a little feng shui meets your personal style and common sense, your home can be transformed from a place where you hang your hat to a magical getaway zone that inspires you each moment you spend at home.

DAY 1: WRITE IT DOWN

Start your retreat in the morning. You'll need a notebook and a pen. Sit up tall, comfortably, wherever you most like to sit in your home. Take a long and deep inhale and exhale. Look around your home and take in what inspires you, and what doesn't. Do you have a favorite painting, object, area of your home that you are drawn to for inspiration? Are there other areas in your home that don't particularly inspire you and that you feel could use a little refresher?

Now close your eyes and begin to rest your attention on your breath. Begin to observe yourself without getting involved emotionally. Do you feel inspired? Do you feel a desire to be inspired? What can you do to

Inspiration from Deepak Chopra

My friend Deepak Chopra always has something original, interesting, soulful, and thoughtful to say. I worked on a project with him that had at its center the theme of transformation. While at the shoot, which was in the beautiful Joshua Tree National Park, the director asked him to talk about motivating people to change their lives. Deepak stopped right there and said, "I don't believe in motivation. I believe in inspiring." He continued to explain that motivation is based on fear, and is not lasting. If you motivate someone it is coming from the outside. For instance: look at that person, don't they motivate you to be better? Don't eat that cookie, motivate yourself to eat broccoli instead. Motivation is forced, pushed, and even if it does work for one instant, it causes stress, builds tension, and is not sustainable.

Inspiration, on the other hand, comes from within and is a lasting, sustainable energy source that is inside of all of us. When we are inspired, we can accomplish anything. There are no limits, no boundaries to our creativity. It's important to inspire ourselves by practicing yoga so we can get connected to our intuition, creativity, and the flow of nature.

change your life so you are more inspired? Open your eyes and write down whatever comes to mind in your notebook. If you have specific ideas about how you would like to re-inspire yourself, write those down, too.

The following are a few ideas to consider incorporating into your home to keep your inspiration flowing. Take them or leave them. I always say in my yoga classes that everything is optional; all you have to do is breathe. If you connect with any of these, run with it; if not, make up your own and have fun.

Power Objects: Don't worry, I'm not talking about displaying anything complicated or scary like a big sword to remind you to take charge of your life; think a bit softer. Do you have anything already lying around your house that makes you feel great when you see it, feel it, smell it? I have a few favorite rocks that I've collected, and a pair of money frogs (little frog figurines that are for good luck and good fortune). If you have a few objects that inspire you, consider putting them together in a corner of a room that feels good to you so you can see them more often.

Good Smells: For a big boost of natural energy and creativity in the morning, try keeping a small bottle of eucalyptus oil by your bedside. Take a whiff of that to get you up feeling refreshed and energized.

Art: You don't have to be a collector of Monet and Van Gogh to be inspired by art in your home. You can even make your own paintings by picking up a blank canvas at an art supply store and a few of your favorite paint colors. Painting can be a great project to inspire you to other endeavors, and when you're finished you'll have something nice to hang on your wall.

Yoga for Inspiration: Morning Routine

Do this routine in the morning either before or after breakfast. If you practice after breakfast, give yourself at least an hour to digest your food before beginning.

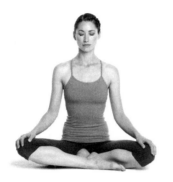

Seated Meditation

Sit up nice and tall, however you can sit most comfortably. Relax your shoulders, so that they are away from your ears. Rest your hands on your thighs. Start to rest your attention on your breath. Watch your inhales come and exhales go. Settle your mind in the space between. Begin to lengthen and deepen your inhales and exhales setting a slow, easy pace of breathing. If a thought starts to enter your mind, simply observe it like a cloud passing by. Continue observing your breath for three to five minutes.

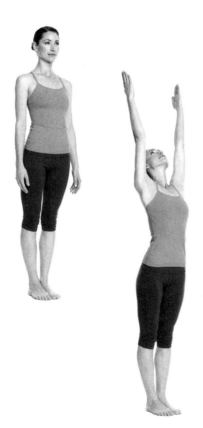

Standing

Stand at the top of your yoga mat. Feet are parallel and slightly apart, under your hip bones. Your hip bones aren't at the outside of your hips so make sure your feet aren't too far apart. You can check by placing two fists between your feet. That's about the width of your hip bones. Close your eyes and bring your attention to your breath. Lengthen and deepen your inhales and exhales and continue breathing at this nice, slow pace for five full breaths. Gently open your eyes.

Standing Arm Reach

Inhale and lift your arms out to your sides and up, filling all the space with your breath and your movement. Relax your tailbone and lift your chest. Keep your shoulders relaxed and down and look up while keeping your face and your forehead relaxed.

Dancer

Shift your weight onto your right leg. Bend your left knee and grab the inside of your left calf with your left hand. Gently press your foot into your hand to open your back. Reach your right arm straight up. Stay here for five long, deep breaths.

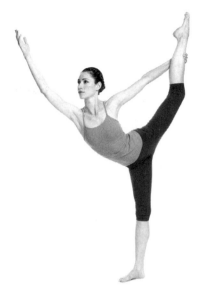

Big Toe Hold

Hug your right knee into your chest and grab your big toe with two fingers of your right hand. Stay here for three long, deep breaths.

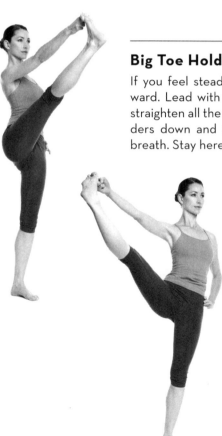

Big Toe Hold with Leg Extended Front

If you feel steady, gently extend your right leg forward. Lead with your heel. If your right leg doesn't straighten all the way, don't force it. Keep your shoulders down and relaxed and stay steady with your breath. Stay here for three long, deep breaths.

Big Toe Hold, Side Extension

From your front extension, open your leg out to your right side. Stay here for three long, deep breaths then bring your leg back to the forward position.

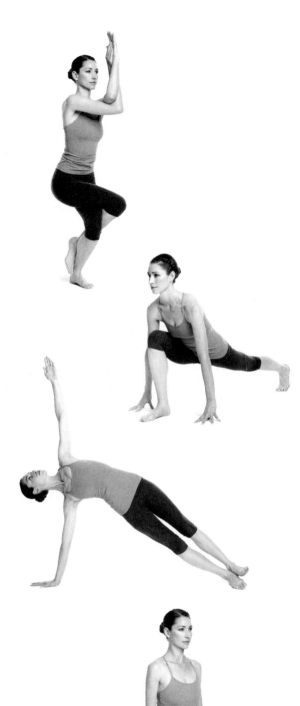

Eagle

From your big toe hold, leg extend side, hug your right knee in toward your chest, bend your left knee, and cross your right leg over your left leg. Hook your foot on either side of your left calf, whichever side feels most comfortable. Wrap your right arm under your left arm. Bend through your left knee and lift up through your arms. Stay here for three long, deep breaths.

Low Lunge

From your eagle, unwind your legs and arms, press your fingertips to the ground and send your left leg back to a low lunge. Sink your hips low. Lengthen out forward through the top of your head and back through your left heel. If it feels good to you, move your body a little side to side and front to back to allow your hips to open up and soften. Stay here for five long, deep breaths.

Side Plank

Press your right palm firmly into the ground. Spread your fingers wide. Lift your hips up, roll to the outside edge of your right foot, and open your hips and torso toward your left. Extend your left arm up and look up toward your left fingers. Stay here for three long, deep breaths and place your left hand on the ground and come to plank.

Up Dog

From your plank, gently lower your knees to the ground, bend your elbows slightly, and drop your shoulders away from your ears. Rock your torso side to side to loosen up any tight areas in your torso. Stay here for three long, deep breaths.

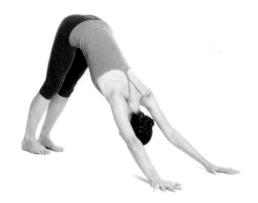

Down Dog

From your up dog, tuck your toes, lift your hips, and press back to down dog. Reach your heels toward the ground. Relax your shoulders and neck toward the ground. Stay here for five long, deep breaths.

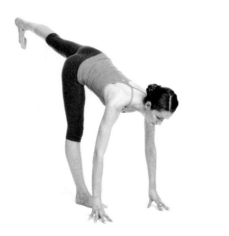

Warrior 3, Fingertips Down

From your down dog, step your right foot forward into a low lunge, shift your weight onto your right leg, and lift your left leg so it's parallel to the ground, keeping your hips square. Press your fingertips into the ground under your shoulders. Stay here for three long, deep breaths.

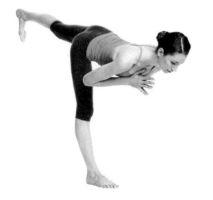

Warrior 3, Palms Press

If you feel steady in warrior 3, try testing your balance by pressing your palms together in front of your chest.

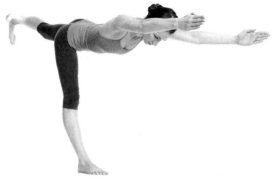

Warrior 3, Straight-Out Arms

If you feel steady with your palms together, try extending your arms straight out in front of you.

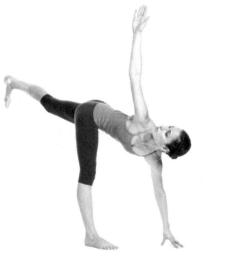

Twisted Half Moon

From your warrior 3, keep your left fingertips under your shoulders and reach your right arm back and up to the ceiling. Twist your torso open toward your right. Extend out evenly from the top of your head through your back heel. Stay here for three long, deep breaths.

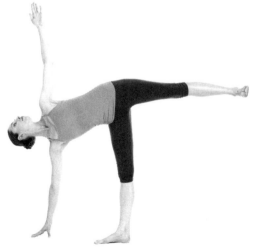

Half Moon

From your twisted half moon, plant your right fingertips down under your right shoulder, open your left hip on top of your right, and open your torso toward your left. Extend your left arm straight up and look up toward your left fingers. Stay here for five long, deep breaths.

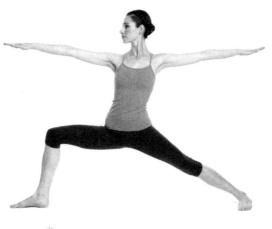

Warrior 2

From your half moon, deeply bend your standing leg, reach your left leg back until your foot meets the ground. Bring your body up to stand and sink your front knee so your front thigh is parallel with the ground. Your hips and torso are open to your left. Open your arms out to the sides in line with your shoulders and gaze over your right fingers. Stay here for five long, deep breaths.

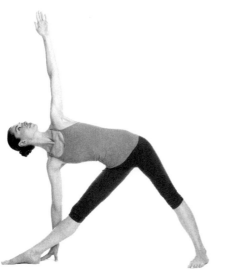

Triangle

From your warrior 2, straighten your right leg so both legs are straight. Lean your torso forward over your front leg, keeping both sides of your torso long. Rest your right hand on your shin or bring your fingertips to the ground if you can. Lean back, open your shoulders, and extend your left arm up above your shoulders. Look up to your left fingers. Stay here for five long, deep breaths.

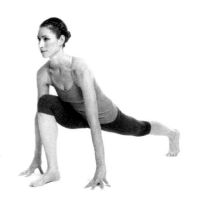

Low Lunge

From your triangle, bend your right knee and press your fingertips on the ground on either side of your front leg, bringing your torso to face forward. Tuck your back toes and straighten your back leg. Sink your hips low. Lengthen out forward through the top of your head and back through your left heel. If it feels good to you, move your body a little side to side and front to back to allow your hips to open up and soften. Stay here for five long, deep breaths.

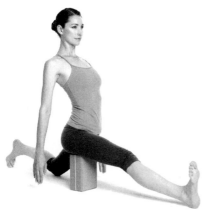

Split (with block)

Grab a block or thick hardcover book. From your low lunge, lower your back knee down to the ground. Flex your front foot and slide your heel out in front of you. Place the block under your right thigh to stabilize your body, if needed. Walk your fingertips back so your shoulders are above your hips. Lift your chest up. Stay here for ten long, deep breaths.

Gently bring yourself out of the split by sitting to the side and making your way back to down dog. Walk your feet up to your hands, roll your torso up to standing, and repeat the whole routine up to this point on the other side.

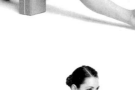
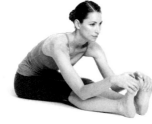

Seated, Both Legs Straight Forward

Sit up tall and bring both legs straight out in front of you. Inhale and lift your arms up. As you exhale, lengthen your torso forward and fold over your legs. If you can't hold the toes easily, bend your knees so your belly can rest on your thighs. You'll get a better opening with bent knees than rounding your back and forcing your hands to your feet. Stay here for ten long, deep breaths.

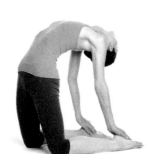

Camel

Kneel, but don't sit, back tall and straight. Inhale and lift your right arm up and back like you are doing the backstroke. If you can grab your right heel easily with your right hand, go for it. If it doesn't happen easily, gently bring yourself back up and do the same on the other side. If you grab your heel easily, swim your other arm up and back to grab hold of your left heel. Lengthen your chest straight up toward the ceiling. Stay here for three long, deep breaths and gently bring your torso upright.

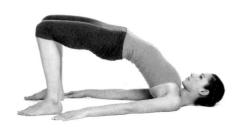

Bridge

Lie down on your back. Bend your knees and press the bottoms of your feet into the ground next to your body so your knees point straight up. Press your arms down by your sides and lift your hips and chest up. Stay here for five long, deep breaths.

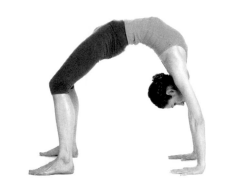

Wheel

Bend your elbows and press your palms into the ground by your ears. Press into your palms firmly and begin to lift the chest up. Straighten your arms only as much as you can while keeping the chest lifted and being able to breathe easily. Lengthen your knees forward and keep your spine long. Stay here for five long, deep breaths. To come down, tuck your chin in toward your chest, bend your elbows, and slowly lower down.

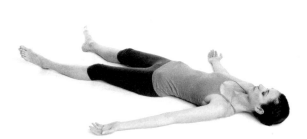

Corpse

Lie down on your back. Open your legs hip width, or a bit wider, depending on what's most comfortable for you. Relax your arms a bit out to your sides, palms facing up. Take a big inhale through your nose, exhale all the air out through your mouth. Repeat the same breathing pattern twice more. Relax your entire self for three to five minutes.

When you are ready to come out of the pose, slowly start to deepen your breath. Roll around your wrists and ankles. Gently hug your knees into your chest and rock up to sit up comfortably.

Go about your day as usual and pay attention to all the little things that provide inspiration in every moment today.

BITES OF BLISS

Whenever I need some inspiration I think spicy. Adding a little kick to your foods gets your system fired up and excited. If you want to keep it simple try adding some red pepper flakes to whatever you're having for dinner. If you're having Mexican or Indian food, try going for the extra spicy version. My favorite do-it-yourself Mexican dish is a spicy black bean and spinach burrito with quinoa instead of rice. Add red pepper and salsa to spice it up! Chai black spice tea is great and you can make it sweet for an after-meal treat by adding a little raw honey.

Yoga for Inspiration: Evening Routine

Do this routine at night either before or after you eat dinner. If you're doing it after dinner, give yourself at least an hour to start digesting your food.

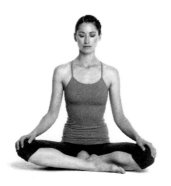

Seated Meditation

Sit up nice and tall, however you can sit most comfortably. Relax your shoulders, so that they are away from your ears. Rest your hands on your thighs (palms up or down, whichever is most comfortable for you). Start to rest your attention on your breath. Watch your inhales come and exhales go. Settle your mind in the space between. Begin to lengthen and deepen your inhales and exhales setting a slow, easy pace of breathing. If a thought starts to enter your mind, simply observe it like a cloud passing by. Let the thought pass and come back to your breath. Continue observing your breath for three to five minutes. A stopwatch could come in handy, or you could simply feel it out and see how much time has actually passed when you open your eyes. Either way is useful.

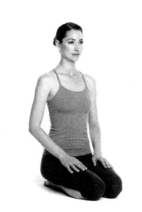

Sit on Heels

Bring yourself onto your knees and sit on your heels. Rest your palms on your thighs, face down. Close your eyes and stay here for ten long, deep breaths.

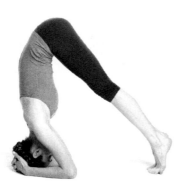

Headstand Prep

Interlace your fingers loosely and place them on the ground. Place the top of your head on the ground so your fingers hold the back of your head. Stay here for a few breaths to get comfortable in the position. Tuck your toes and straighten your legs as you would in a down dog. In this position you are getting a lot of the benefits of a headstand without your feet even leaving the ground. Stay here for ten long, deep breaths and when you are ready to come out of it gently lower your knees to the ground and relax in child's pose.

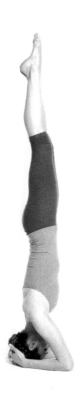

Headstand

Start to walk your feet in toward your body so your hips line up over your shoulders and your back is vertical. Stay here for a few breaths. Bend one knee in and bring your heel to your hip. Bring it back down and try the other leg. Try both legs at the same time. When your heels are pulled in toward your hips, slowly extend your legs straight up. Stay for twenty long, deep breaths if you can. When you are ready to come down, slowly lower one leg at a time and rest in child's pose for a few breaths.

Bridge

Lie down on your back. Bend your knees and press the bottoms of your feet into the ground next to your body so your knees point straight up. Press your arms down by your sides and lift your hips and chest up. Stay here for five long, deep breaths.

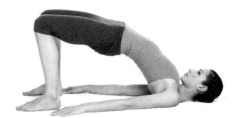

Wheel

Bend your elbows and press your palms into the ground by your ears. Press into your palms firmly and begin to lift the chest up. Straighten your arms only as much as you can while keeping the chest lifted and being able to breathe easily. Lengthen your knees forward and keep your spine long. Stay here for five long, deep breaths. To come down, tuck your chin in toward your chest, bend your elbows, and slowly lower down.

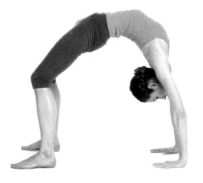

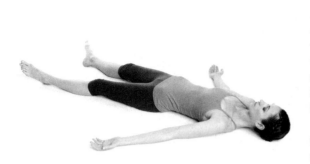

Corpse

Lie down on your back. Open your legs hip width, or a bit wider, depending on what's most comfortable for you. Relax your arms a bit out to your sides, palms facing up. Take a big inhale through your nose, exhale all the air out through your mouth. Repeat the same breathing pattern twice more. Relax your entire self for three to five minutes.

When you are ready to come out of it, slowly start to deepen your breath. Roll your wrists and ankles around. Gently hug your knees into your chest and rock up to sit up comfortably.

Try to keep distractions to a minimum before bedtime. Read a book that you've been putting off starting, or journal instead of watching TV or using the computer. Keep a notebook by your bed in case you want to write down any inspirational thoughts. Sleep well!

DAY 2: WAKE AND REFLECT

When you wake in the morning, sit up in bed and lean against the wall or a headboard if you have one. Relax your hands on your thighs and pay attention to your breath. Stay here and meditate for a few minutes. When you are finished, write down in your journal anything that comes to mind, anything at all. If you have any thoughts about Day 1 of the retreat, write them down also.

Before breakfast, do the morning routine. Go about your day as usual doing what you need to get done, keep drinking lots of water, and making healthy choices. If you'd like to stay in "retreat mode" for the day, pick a fun activity that inspires you, whether that's picking up a paintbrush or guitar, going for a nature walk, or heading to the nearest art gallery.

At night, before dinner, set aside ten minutes for meditation. Keep your journal handy. Write down any thoughts or inspirations that are on your mind. Sit up tall, comfortably, wherever you most like to sit in your home. Take a long and deep inhale and exhale. Close your eyes and rest your attention on your breath. If your mind starts to wander, gently guide it back to your breath. If you think of something inspiring and you don't want to lose the thought, write it down and come back to your meditation.

Go about your day as usual and be on the lookout for spontaneous inspiration!

Do the evening routine either before or after dinner. When it is time for bed, again try to avoid the overstimulation of TV or staring at a computer screen. You may think these things calm you, but they really don't. Read or write in your journal before bed. Keep it and a big glass of water by your bed. When you wake in the morning repeat the morning meditation and journal writing. This time after you've written whatever first comes to mind, write about your experience over the last two days. If there is any part of the retreat you found useful that you can integrate into your daily life, write it down with the intention of doing so.

Relax, Restore, and Rejuvenate Retreat

Our lives can get so hectic that having a calm, comfortable space where we can completely let go and unwind is essential. Our homes should be a place where we feel at peace and can relax fully. This retreat is designed to relax, restore, and rejuvenate you completely right from the comfort of your own home . . . which is a lot cheaper than a spa!

DAY 1: WRITE IT DOWN AND WIND IT DOWN

Start your retreat in the evening. You'll need a blanket, a notebook, and a pen. Sit up tall and comfortably, wherever you most like to sit in your home. Take a long, deep breath in and out. Look around your home and take in what helps you relax and unwind and what doesn't. Is there anything that you can adjust slightly that will aid in your rejuvenation at home? Maybe tossing a blanket over the couch or clearing space around your bed for your yoga practice would help.

What else? Sit on it and think a bit. Then do this routine.

Yoga for Relaxation: Evening Routine

Try to keep distractions to a minimum before bedtime. Read a book or journal instead of watching TV or using the computer. Keep a journal or notebook by your bed in case you want to write down any thoughts. Sleep well!

Reclining Butterfly

Roll up a blanket tightly, like a burrito. Sit up and place the blanket behind your hips, perpendicular to them. Roll down on the blanket so it's lined up under your spine. Bring the bottoms of your feet together and relax your knees out to the sides. Stay here for three to five minutes. Allow your breath to shift to long and deep. Focus on your exhales a bit more than the inhales to further promote relaxation. When you're ready to come out of the pose, gently roll onto your right side and press your hands into the floor to bring you back to sitting.

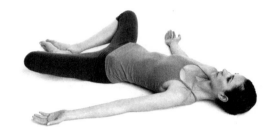

BITES OF BLISS

To help promote a restful night's sleep try drinking a bedtime tea. Anything that has chamomile, peppermint, or spearmint is great to help you get to sleep, stay asleep, and wake up feeling refreshed and energized. Valerian root is also a natural sleep aid that you can find in tea form. Drink it sparingly. Large doses or overuse may result in stomachache or mild depression.

WAKE AND REFLECT

When you wake in the morning, sit up in bed and lean against the wall or a headboard if you have one. Relax your hands on your thighs and pay attention to your breath. Stay here and meditate for a few minutes. When you are finished, write down in your journal anything that comes to mind. If you feel rested, or not, write it down.

Restorative Yoga: Morning Routine

Do this routine in the morning either before or after breakfast. If you do eat breakfast, allow yourself about an hour to digest your meal before you do the routine.

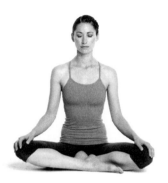

Seated Meditation

Sit up nice and tall, however you can sit most comfortably. Relax your shoulders, so that they are away from your ears. Rest your hands on your thighs. Start to rest your attention on your breath. Watch your inhales come and exhales go. Settle your mind in the space between. Begin to lengthen and deepen your inhales and exhales setting a slow, easy pace of breathing. If a thought starts to enter your mind, simply observe it like a cloud passing by. Continue observing your breath for three to five minutes.

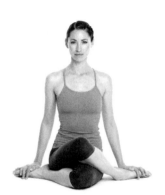

Cow Face

Start seated, however you can sit without pain. It can be on a pillow or on the floor if it's easy for you. Press your hands into the ground on either side of your knees, and bring yourself to a kneeling position, supporting your weight with your hands on the ground. Bring your right knee in front of your left knee so they are directly in a line. Move your feet out to the sides. Gently sit your hips back either to the ground or to the floor. Your knees will now be stacked on top of each other. If there is tension in the knees or hips bring a pillow or a block under your hips to allow more room for your hips and knees to open without stress. Sit in a straight line, shoulders directly aligned with your hips. Rest your hands near your feet. Lift your chest so that the muscles feel open and your shoulders are back, and sit up tall. Stay here for ten long, deep breaths.

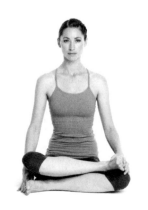

Seated Ankle to Knee

Sit up tall. Bend your knees in and stack your right leg on top of your left leg so your right ankle is on top of your left knee and your right knee is on top of your left ankle. Stay here for ten long, deep breaths. Then repeat with the other leg.

Pigeon

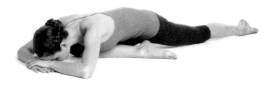

From your ankle to knee, lean into your right hip and reach your left leg long behind you. If your hips don't reach the ground sit on a pillow or a block. Turn your hips and shoulders so they both face forward. Stay here for ten long, deep breaths.

Do the whole routine up until this point on the other side, beginning with cow face pose.

Bridge on Block

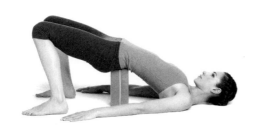

Have a block handy. Lie down, bend your knees in, and place your feet on the ground next to your body so your knees point straight up. Lift your hips and place the block under your lower back. This should feel good so adjust the block accordingly. The block can be higher or lower depending on how you turn it. Stay here for twenty long, deep breaths.

Corpse

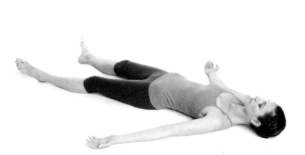

Lie down on your back. Open your legs hip width, or a bit wider, depending on what's most comfortable for you. Relax your arms a bit out to your sides, palms facing up. Take a big inhale through your nose, exhale all the air out through your mouth. Repeat the same breathing pattern twice more. Relax your entire self for three to five minutes.

When you are ready to come out of it, slowly start to deepen your breath. Roll your wrists and ankles around. Gently hug your knees into your chest and rock up to sit up comfortably.

Go about your day as usual and try to stay as relaxed as possible, even when completing everyday tasks.

Day 2
Restorative Yoga: Evening Routine

Try the routine after a bath for optimal relaxation.

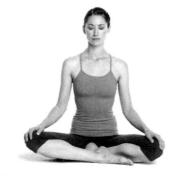

Seated Meditation

Sit up nice and tall, however you can sit most comfortably. Relax your shoulders, so that they are away from your ears. Rest your hands on your thighs. Start to rest your attention on your breath. Watch your inhales come and exhales go. Settle your mind in the space between. Begin to lengthen and deepen your inhales and exhales setting a slow, easy pace of breathing. If a thought starts to enter your mind, simply observe it like a cloud passing by. Continue observing your breath for three to five minutes.

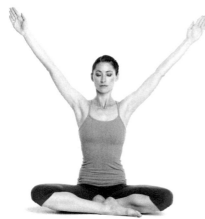

Seated Meditation Arms in V

Staying in your comfortable seated position, raise your arms overhead so they are in a V shape. Relax your shoulders downward and reach out through your fingertips. This may not seem like anything at first but we are going to stay and breathe here for three minutes. Practicing meditation with your arms up like this adds a level of intensity that will help you relax once you get past the discomfort from keeping your arms up. Finding the ease in staying here for several minutes will clear your mind and release loads of tension from your body.

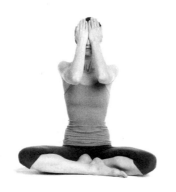

Calm Eyes

Sit up nice and tall, however you can sit comfortably. Rub the palms of your hands together pretty quickly to get a good amount of heat going. Close your eyes and gently press the heels of your hands into your eyelids. Rest your fingers against your forehead. Stay here for three long, deep breaths and gently relax your hands to rest on your thighs.

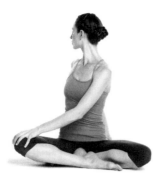

Seated Easy Twist

From your comfortable seated position, inhale and lift your left arm up. As you exhale, rest your left hand on your right knee. Press your right fingertips into the ground behind your hips. Inhale and lengthen your torso up tall. Exhale and twist your torso around to the right.

Seated, Arms Crossed Hold Knees

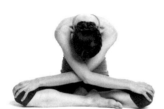

From your seated easy twist, inhale your right arm up and over your body and grab hold of your left knee, so both hands are holding opposite knees. Relax your head and neck. Stay here for three long, deep breaths and gently roll your torso upright. Do the same thing on the other side.

Plow

Extend your legs forward and roll down to lie on your back. Press your arms down by your sides, round your back, and bring your feet over your head into a plow pose.

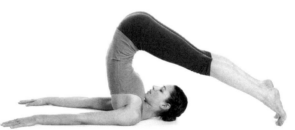

Shoulder Stand

If your neck feels pretty tight in your plow, stay there a little longer and then slowly roll back down to lie on your back. If your neck feels good in your plow, press your palms into your back so your fingers face up. Wiggle your elbows closer together and scoot your hands up your back close to your shoulders. Lift the backs of your legs straight up so your body is in one straight line. Stay here for twenty long, deep breaths. Either close your eyes or keep your gaze softly resting on your belly button.

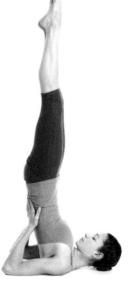

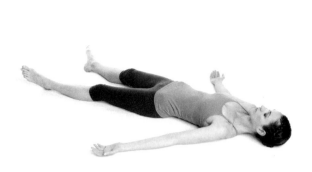

Corpse

Lie down on your back. Open your legs hip width, or a bit wider, depending on what's most comfortable for you. Relax your arms a bit out to your sides, palms facing up. Take a big inhale through your nose, exhale all the air out through your mouth. Repeat the same breathing pattern twice more. Relax your entire self for three to five minutes.

When you are ready to come out of it, slowly start to deepen your breath. Roll your wrists and ankles around. Gently hug your knees into your chest and rock up to sit up comfortably.

After you've finished your nightly yoga, tuck yourself in. Keep your journal handy if you want to write anything down that comes to mind and sleep well!

Just a Few More Thoughts Before You Close This Book

My hope is that whether you are at the beginning of your efforts to fit yoga and healthy living ideas into your life or are already a longtime yoga practitioner, teacher, guide, master, or fall somewhere in between, you are inspired to practice and share yoga with everyone you know and care about. As I've said a lot in this book, tailor yoga to work for your life, around your needs, and to achieve your goals, as yoga is for everyone. I hope you claim it, make it as natural as waking up every day, and as routine as drinking a glass of water. I hope you take wild advantage of the fact that yoga really does cure.

A regular yoga practice is entirely what you make of it. You don't have to be able—or even want—to put your foot behind your head or hang out in the splits to gain its incredible transformative benefits. Those who practice yoga regularly will enjoy tremendous health and vitality, boundless energy, and an increased zest for life. Yoga also shows us how to become sensitized to our needs, our wants, and our selves, and builds the intuition we need to deal with stress, ailments, and any of the curveballs life tosses our way.

Yoga shows us how to be easy and calm, no matter the circumstance. And for the situations that yoga doesn't cure, a regular practice helps us to deal with them with grace and ease.

Whether shown through the efforts of researchers, personal stories of transformation, or every day practices and ideas that have been passed down through the centuries, yoga is as natural in our lives as breathing. We already have within us everything we need to live an inspired, healthy life full of vitality and zest for each moment. It's simply up to us what we do with what we have.

Your life does matter. Your contribution does matter. Anything is possible.

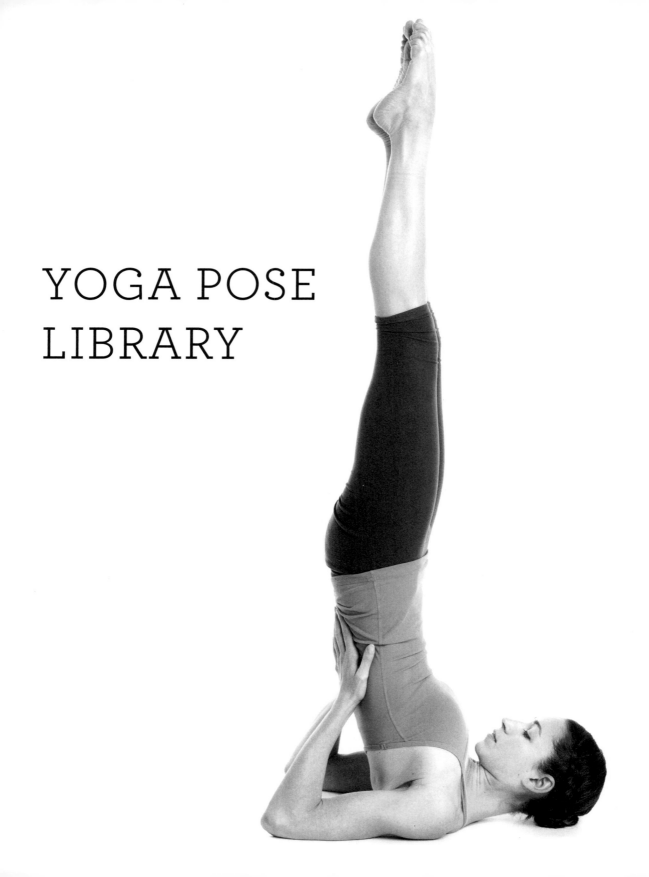

YOGA POSE
LIBRARY

The yoga poses compiled here were created by experimentation over the years to focus the practitioner inward to heal the body and mind.

Whether you practice for health reasons, mental clarity, spiritual connection, or all of the above, you can tailor yoga to your lifestyle, intentions, and goals. Remember to breathe, be easy on yourself, and most of all, enjoy. The practice of yoga allows us to experience our whole selves. It's up to us what we do with that experience.

This index includes some of the major benefits of each pose. Remember to breathe long and deeply. Namaste!

Standing Poses

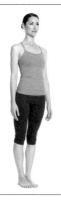

1. Standing. Improves posture, confidence, and body awareness.

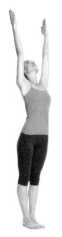

2. Standing Arm Reach (Sun Salutation). Improves posture and expands the lungs.

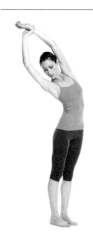

3. Standing Side Opener (wrist pull). Improves posture and expands the lungs.

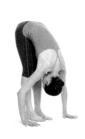

4. Standing Forward Bend. Calms the mind, opens the hamstrings, and releases tension in the upper back.

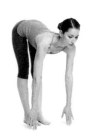

5. Standing Forward Bend (flat back arch) (Sun Salutations). Lengthens the spine and opens the hamstrings.

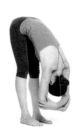

6. Standing Forward Bend (elbow hold). Opens the hamstrings, calms the mind, and releases tension in the upper back.

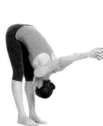

7. Standing Forward Bend (shoulder opener). Opens the hamstrings and shoulders, and calms the mind.

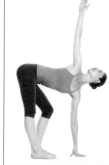

8. Back Lengthener Easy Twist. Lengthens the spine and opens the hamstrings.

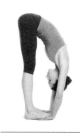

9. Standing Forward Bend (step on hands). Releases the wrists, opens the hamstrings, and calms the mind.

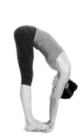

10. Standing Forward Bend (step on palms). Releases the wrists, opens the hamstrings, and calms the mind.

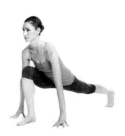

11. Low Lunge.
Opens the hips and lengthens the spine.

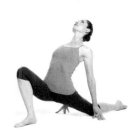

12. Low Lunge (back knee down, arch).
Opens the hips and lengthens the spine.

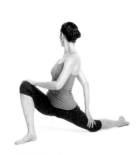

13. Low Lunge (back knee down, twist).
Opens the hips, lengthens the spine, and promotes blood flow to the vital organs.

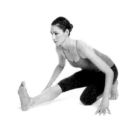

14. Runner's Stretch.
Opens the hamstrings and calms the mind.

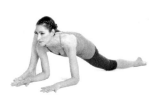

15. Lizard.
Opens the hips and releases emotional tension.

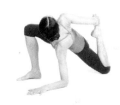

16. Lizard Twist (ankle hold). Opens the hips and spine.

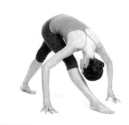

17. Single Leg Forward Bend.
Opens the hamstrings, lengthens the spine, and calms the mind.

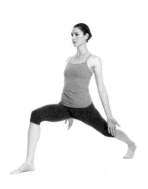

18. High Lunge (arms down).
Builds body awareness, builds strength in the legs, and improves balance.

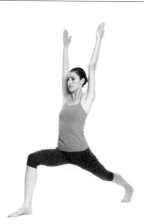

19. High Lunge (arms up). Builds body awareness, builds strength in the legs, opens the torso, and improves balance.

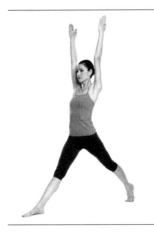

20. High Lunge (arms and hips up). Builds body awareness, builds strength in the legs, opens the torso, and improves balance and coordination.

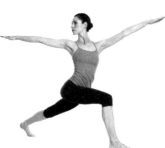

21. High Lunge Twist. Promotes blood flow to the vital organs, and builds strength in the hips, hamstrings, shoulders, and arms.

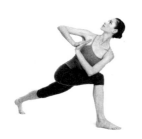

22. High Lunge Prayer Twist. Promotes blood flow to the vital organs, tones the abdominals, and strengthens the legs.

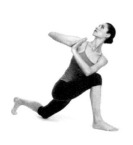

23. High Lunge Prayer Twist (back knee down). Promotes blood flow to the vital organs, tones the abdominals, and calms the mind.

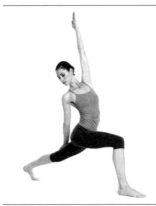

24. High Lunge Twist Reverse. Strengthens the legs, and improves balance and coordination.

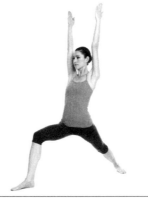

25. Warrior 1. Strengthens the legs, opens the hips, and builds confidence.

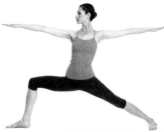

26. Warrior 2. Strengthens the legs, opens the hips, and builds confidence.

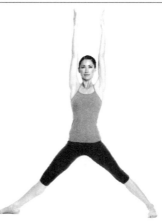

27. Warrior 2 (arms up, legs straight). Strengthens the legs, open the hips, and expands the lungs.

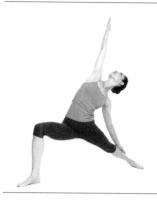

28. Reverse Warrior. Strengthens the legs, opens the hips, lengthens the torso, and expands the lungs.

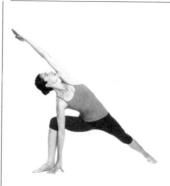

32. Extended Angle (fingertips down). Strengthens the legs, opens the torso and shoulders, and expands the lungs.

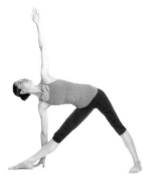

29. Triangle. Improves body awareness, strengthens the legs, and lengthens the torso.

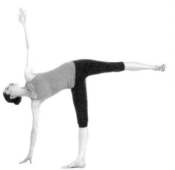

33. Half Moon. Improves body awareness and balance, strengthens the legs, and opens the torso.

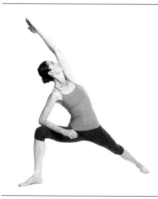

30. Extended Angle (forearm on thigh). Strengthens the legs, lengthens the torso, and opens the spine.

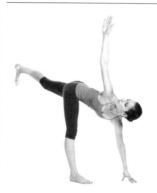

34. Twisted Half Moon. Improves body awareness and balance, strengthens the legs, and improves blood flow to the vital organs.

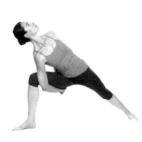

31. Extended Angle Bind. Strengthens the legs, opens the torso and shoulders, and improves concentration.

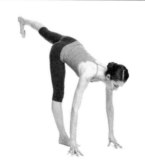

35. Warrior 3 (fingertips down). Strengthens the legs, lengthens the torso, and improves body awareness and balance.

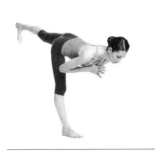

36. Warrior 3 (palms press). Strengthens the legs, lengthens the torso, and improves body awareness and balance.

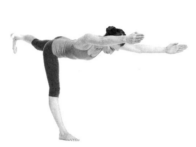

37. Warrior 3 (straight out arms). Strengthens the legs, lengthens the torso, and improves body awareness, balance, and concentration.

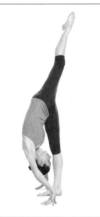

38. Standing Split. Strengthens the legs, opens the legs, releases tension in the head and neck, and calms the mind.

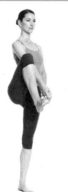

39. Big Toe Hold. Strengthens the legs, improves balance, and builds concentration.

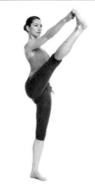

40. Big Toe Hold (leg extend front). Strengthens the legs, improves balance, improves flexibility, and builds concentration.

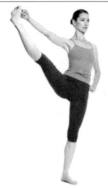

41. Big Toe Hold (leg extend side). Strengthens the legs, improves balance, improves flexibility, and builds concentration.

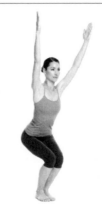

42. Chair. Strengthens the legs, lengthens the torso, and improves concentration.

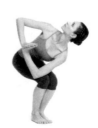

43. Chair Twist. Strengthens the legs, lengthens the torso, improves concentration, and improves blood flow to the vital organs.

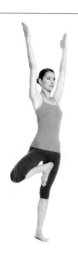

44. Tree (arms up). Strengthens the legs, and improves balance and concentration.

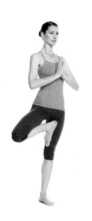

45. Tree (arms prayer). Strengthens the legs, and improves balance and concentration.

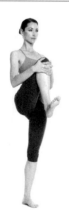

46. Standing Shin Hug. Strengthens the legs, and improves balance and concentration.

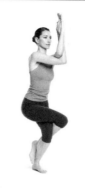

47. Eagle. Strengthens the legs, and improves balance and concentration.

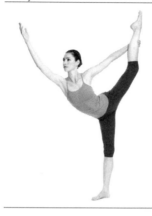

48. Dancer. Strengthens the legs, and improves flexibility, balance, and concentration.

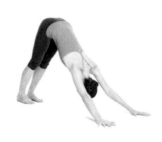

49. Down Dog. Opens the backs of the legs, opens the shoulders, releases tension in the head and neck, improves blood flow in the entire body, and calms the mind.

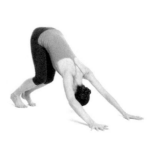

50. Down Dog (bend knees and elbows). Opens the backs of the legs more gently than down dog, opens the shoulders, releases tension in the head and neck, improves blood flow in the entire body, and calms the mind.

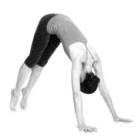

51. Down Dog (lift heels). Opens the backs of the legs, strengthens the calves, releases tension in the head and neck, improves blood flow in the entire body, and calms the mind.

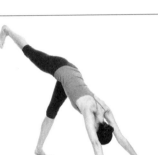

52. Down Dog Split. Improves flexibility in the hamstrings, releases tension in the head and neck, improves blood flow in the entire body, improves circulation in the legs, and calms the mind.

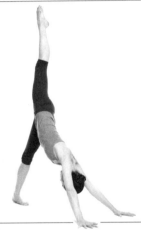

53. Down Dog Split (open hips). Improves range of motion in the hips, improves flexibility in the hamstrings, releases tension in the head and neck, improves blood flow in the entire body, improves circulation in the legs, and calms the mind.

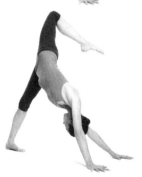

54. Down Dog Split (open hips, bent knee). Improves range of motion in the hips, improves flexibility in the hamstrings, opens the torso, releases tension in the head and neck, improves circulation in the legs, and calms the mind.

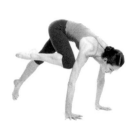

55. Down Dog (knee to elbow). Improves body awareness, strengthens the abdominals, strengthens the arms, strengthens the legs, and improves concentration.

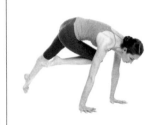

56. Down Dog (split knee across). Improves body awareness, strengthens the abdominals, strengthens the arms, strengthens the legs, improves concentration and balance, and promotes blood flow to the vital organs.

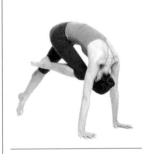

57. Down Dog (split knee to nose). Improves body awareness, strengthens the abdominals, strengthens the arms and legs, and improves concentration.

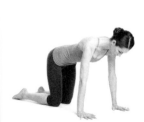

58. Hands and Knees Neutral Spine. Calms the mind and improves body awareness.

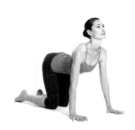

59. Cow.
Opens the spine and calms the mind.

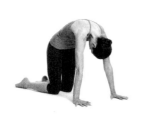

60. Cat.
Opens the spine and calms the mind.

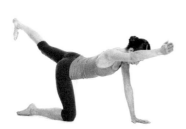

61. Hands and Knees (opposite leg and arm extend). Builds body awareness, and strengthens the legs, arms, and abdominals.

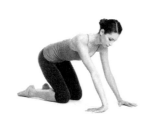

62. Hands and Knees (wrist release). Releases tension in the wrists.

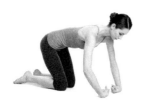

63. Hands and Knees (fist release). Releases tension in the wrists.

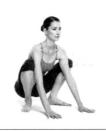

64. Squat.
Opens the hips and calms the mind.

65. Squat (neck release). Opens the hips, releases tension in the neck, and calms the mind.

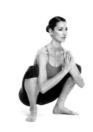

66. Squat (palm press). Opens the hips and opens the spine.

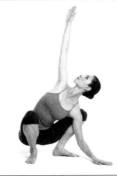

67. Squat (open arm twist). Opens the hips, lengthens the spine, and opens the shoulders.

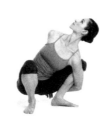

68. Squat Twist Bind. Opens the hips, lengthens the spine, and improves range of motion in the shoulders.

Seated Poses

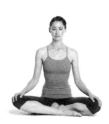

69. Seated Meditation. Opens the hips, lengthens the spine, improves posture, gets you connected, and calms and opens the mind.

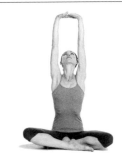

73. Seated Palm Press. Opens the hips and lengthens the torso.

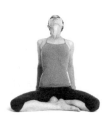

70. Seated Chest Lift (fingertips behind tail bone). Opens the hips, lengthens the spine, and opens the chest.

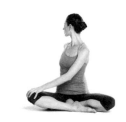

74. Seated Easy Twist (hand on opposite knee). Opens the hips, shoulders, torso, and improves digestion and blood flow to the vital organs.

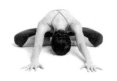

71. Seated Easy Forward Bend (cross-legged). Opens the hips and calms the mind.

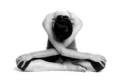

75. Seated arm cross hold knees (cross-legged). Opens the hips, and releases tension in the neck and head.

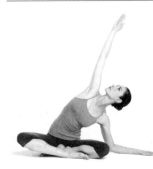

72. Seated Easy Side Bend (cross-legged, forearm lower). Opens the hips and lengthens the torso.

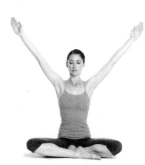

76. Seated Meditation (arms in V). Opens the hips, improves concentration, and calms and opens the mind.

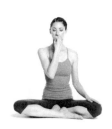

77. Alternate Nostril Breathing. Regulates the nervous system, calms the mind, and improves breathing and lung capacity.

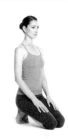

82. Sit on Heels (toes tucked). Lengthens the spine, and opens the arches of the feet.

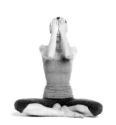

78. Calm Eyes. Eases eye tension and calms the mind.

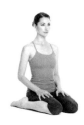

83. Hero. Improves posture and aids digestion.

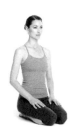

79. Sit on Heels (palms in lap). Lengthens the spine, improves posture, and calms the mind.

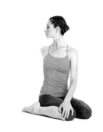

84. Hero Twist. Improves posture, aids digestion, and promotes blood flow to the vital organs.

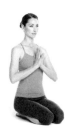

80. Sit on Heels (palms together). Lengthens the spine, improves posture, and calms the mind.

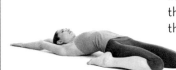

85. Hero (reclined). Opens up the spine, improves health of the knees, and calms the mind.

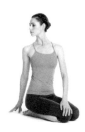

81. Sit on Heels Easy Twist. Lengthens the spine, and improves blood flow to the vital organs.

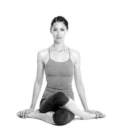

86. Cow Face. Opens the hips and calms the mind.

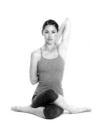

87. Cow Face with Shoulder Opener (upright). Opens up the hips and shoulders, and calms the mind.

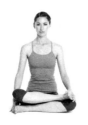

88. Cow Face with Shoulder Opener (forward bend). Opens up the hips and shoulders, lengthens the spine, and calms the mind.

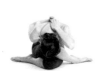

89. Ankle to Knee. Opens up the hips and calms the mind.

90. Ankle to Knee (forward bend). Opens up the hips and calms the mind.

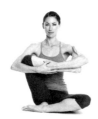

91. Seated Shin Hug. Releases tension in the hips and improves range of motion in the hip joint.

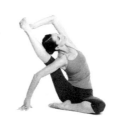

92. Compass. Releases tension in the hips and hamstrings, and improves range of motion in the hip joint.

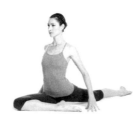

93. Pigeon (upright). Releases tension in the hips.

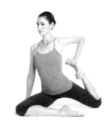

94. Pigeon (front of thigh release). Releases tension in the hips and front of thighs.

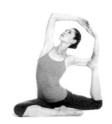

95. Pigeon (full). Releases tension in the hips and thighs, and opens the spine.

96. Pigeon (torso release). Releases tension in the hips, lengthens the torso, and calms the mind.

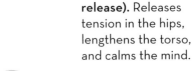

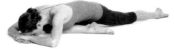

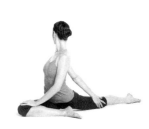

97. Pigeon Twist.
Releases tension in the hips, opens the spine, and aids digestion.

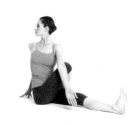

102. Seated Spine Twist (one leg straight). Lengthens the spine and improves blood flow to the vital organs.

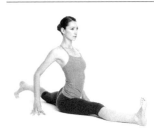

98. Splits.
Releases tension in the hips, improves flexibility in the hamstrings, and calms the mind.

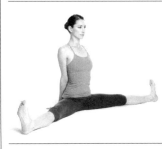

103. Seated Wide Leg Straddle (torso upright). Opens the hips and hamstrings.

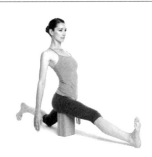

99. Splits with Block.
Releases tension in the hips, improves flexibility in the hamstrings, and calms the mind.

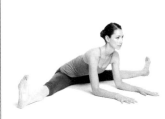

104. Seated Wide Leg Straddle (torso lower). Opens the hips, hamstrings, and spine.

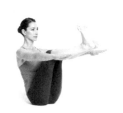

100. Boat.
Strengthens the abdominals and builds concentration.

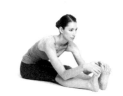

105. Seated Both Legs Straight Forward Bend. Opens the hamstrings, lengthens the spine, and calms the mind.

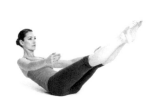

101. Half Boat.
Strengthens the abdominals and builds concentration.

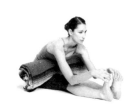

106. Seated Both Legs Straight Forward Bend (blanket on lap). Calms the mind and gently opens the hamstrings.

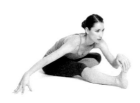

107. Seated One Leg Forward Bend. Opens the hamstrings and lower back.

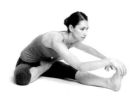

108. Seated One Leg Forward Bend (foot on hip crease). Opens the hamstrings and lower back, and aids digestion.

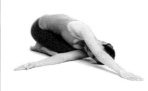

109. Child's Pose Twist. Releases tension in the shoulders and calms the mind.

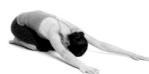

110. Child's Pose. Cools the body and calms the mind.

Backbends

111. Up Dog.
Opens the spine and energizes the mind.

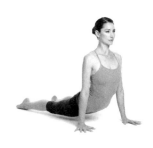

112. Knees Chest Chin (Sun Salutation).
Opens the spine and improves body awareness.

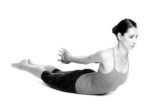

113. Lying on Stomach (interlace hands behind back, opener).
Opens the spine and invigorates the mind.

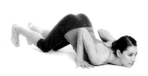

114. Bow.
Opens the spine and hips, and invigorates the mind.

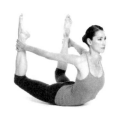

115. Camel Swim.
Opens the spine and hips, and energizes the whole body.

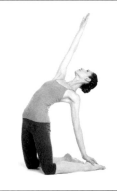

116. Camel.
Opens the spine and hips, and energizes the whole body.

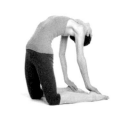

117. Bridge Prep.
Opens the spine, releases tension in the upper back, and invigorates the mind.

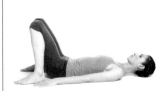

118. Bridge.
Opens the spine, releases tension in the upper back, and invigorates the mind.

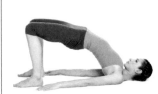

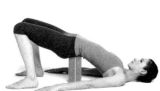

119. Bridge (interlace hands). Opens the spine, releases tension in the shoulders, and invigorates the mind.

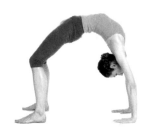

121. Wheel. Opens the spine and invigorates the mind.

120. Bridge with Block. Opens the spine and calms the mind.

Inversions and Arm Balances

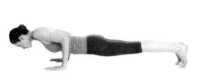

122. Plank. Strengthens the entire body and improves concentration.

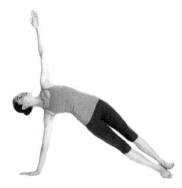

123. Plank Push-up. Strengthens the entire body and improves concentration.

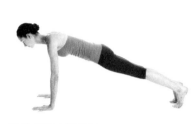

124. Side Plank. Builds body awareness, opens up the sides of the torso, and improves concentration.

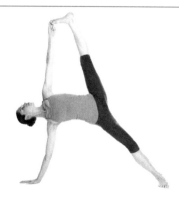

125. Side Plank with Leg Extend. Builds body awareness, opens up the hamstrings, and improves concentration.

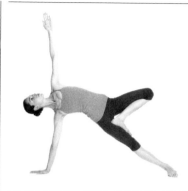

126. Side Plank Tree. Builds body awareness, opens up the sides of the torso, and improves balance.

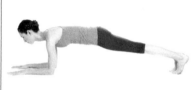

127. Forearm Plank. Builds body awareness, strengthens the shoulders, and improves balance.

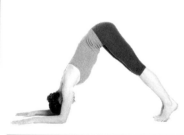

128. Forearm Stand Prep (Down Dog). Builds body awareness, strengthens the shoulders, and improves balance.

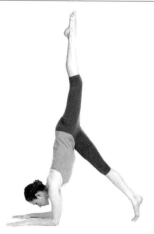

129. Forearm Stand Prep (lift leg). Builds body awareness, strengthens the shoulders, and improves coordination.

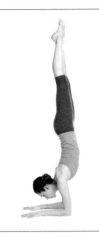

130. Forearm Stand.
Builds body awareness, improves focus, strengthens the shoulders, and improves balance.

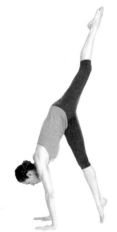

131. Handstand Rocks.
Builds body awareness, improves focus, strengthens the shoulders, and improves balance.

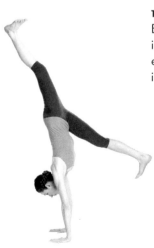

132. Handstand L Shape.
Builds body awareness, improves focus, strengthens the shoulders, and improves balance.

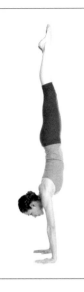

133. Handstand.
Builds body awareness, improves focus, strengthens the shoulders, and improves balance.

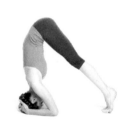

134. Headstand Prep (feet on ground).

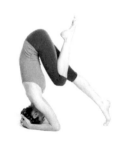

135. Headstand Prep (one foot to hip).

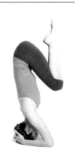

136. Headstand Prep (both feet to hips).

137. Headstand.
Calms the mind, sharpens focus, and improves circulation.

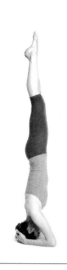

138. Crow.
Builds body awareness and confidence, and strengthens the abdominals and arms.

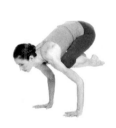

139. Side Crow.
Builds body awareness and confidence, and strengthens the abdominals and arms.

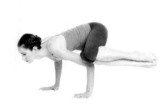

140. Plow. Releases tension in the neck and upper back, and calms the mind.

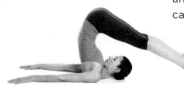

141. Legs Up the Wall.
Improves circulation and eases the mind.

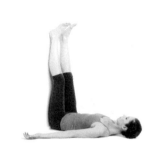

142. Supported Shoulder Stand (with block).
Improves circulation and eases the mind.

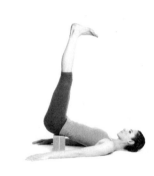

143. Shoulder Stand.
Improves posture, regulates thyroid function, improves circulation, corrects imbalance in the nervous system, sharpens the mind, and relaxes the brain.

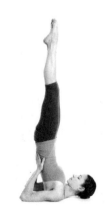

Reclining

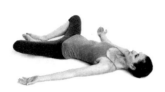

144. Reclined Butterfly. Opens the spine and hips, and improves creativity.

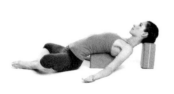

145. Reclined Butterfly spine opener (with blankets). Opens the spine, releases tension in the hips, and releases emotional stress.

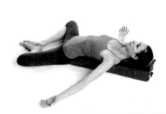

146. Reclined Butterfly Spine Opener (with blocks). Opens the spine, releases tension in the hips, and releases emotional stress.

147. Reclined Straight Legs Spine Opener(with blocks). Opens the spine, releases tension in the hips and lower back, and releases emotional tension.

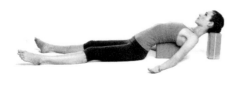

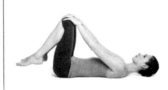

148. Reclining Hold (knees). Releases tension in the back and hips, and calms the mind.

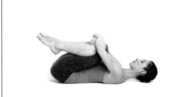

149. Reclined Single Knee Hug. Releases tension in the hips and calms the mind.

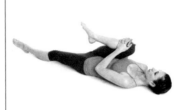

150. Reclining Knee Hug. Releases tension in the back and hips.

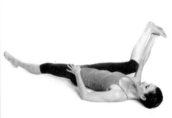

151. Half Happy Baby. Releases tension in the hips and back, and releases emotional stress.

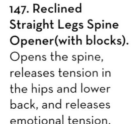

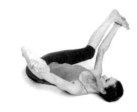

152. Happy Baby. Releases tension in the hips and back, and releases emotional stress.

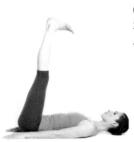

153. Leg Raises (feet straight up). Strengthens the back and abdominals.

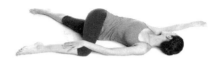

156. Reclined Single Knee Hug Twist. Releases tension in the spine and calms the mind.

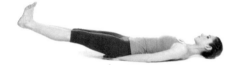

154. Leg Raises (feet lower). Strengthens the back and abdominals.

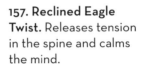

157. Reclined Eagle Twist. Releases tension in the spine and calms the mind.

155. Reclining Hamstring Release. Releases tension in the hamstrings.

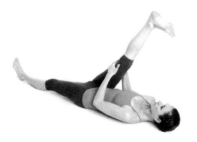

158. Corpse. Relaxes the entire body and mind deeply.

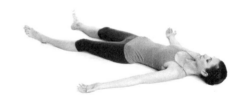

Acknowledgments

So many fantastic people who I have the good fortune of knowing have transformed what I do from something in my head into something I can share, see, and hold in my hands. Our interrelated lives continue to inspire me daily.

Thank you, Will Hobbs, for considering my ambitions in so many of your daily interactions. It's not a small task. Heather Jackson, this book simply would not exist without you. You are an angel and a wizard and I am truly grateful that you have offered up and shared with me your plethora of talents, sharp eye, rich brain, and incredibly determined sensibilities. I admire you so much and my hope is that this is just the beginning. Heather Lazare, thank you for believing in and getting excited about *Yoga Cures* and welcoming me into the fold at Crown so warmly. Amanda Patten, thank you for your warm enthusiasm and sharp set of eyes and sensibilities. Kelsey Robinson, Catherine Pollack, Jonathan Lazzara, Stephanie Knapp, Ellen Folan, Rosalie Wieder, and the Random House team, thank you for your guidance and inspired support. Simon Green, thank you for your efforts and patience. Durk Snowden, Heidi Kristoffer, Faith Smith, Leslie Lewis, Todd Belt, Dave, and everyone who shared their *Yoga Cures* story with me, you are all so touching and inspiring. Michael, our daily life cultivates and refines the language I use to communicate this stuff, so thank you. Deepak, you've shared and given me so much, so freely. How did I get so lucky?

About the Author

Named "Yoga Rebel" by the *New York Times*, Tara Stiles has inspired a wide audience around the world with her healthy and relatable approach to yoga, meditation, exercise, awareness, nutrition, and everyday well-being. Tara has been featured in publications including *Elle, Lucky, In-Style, Esquire,* and *Men's Health,* and has been profiled by several national and international papers including the *Times of India, The Times* (UK), and Sweden's *Dagens Nyheter.*

Tara is the founder and owner of Strala Yoga, widely known for its unpretentious, inclusive, and straightforward approach to yoga and healthy living. She is the personal yoga instructor to Deepak Chopra, whom she's collaborated with to create the Authentic Yoga app, as well as the Yoga Transformation DVD series among other projects. Jane Fonda named Tara "the new face of fitness." They partnered to relaunch Jane's famous *Workout* brand of fitness DVDs and equipment.

Tara is the author of *Slim Calm Sexy Yoga.* Her approach leads people to their own intuition and awareness. The results are radiant health and lasting happiness. As *Vanity Fair* noted, "Tara Stiles has got to be the coolest yoga instructor ever."